T0061805

Contents

Praise for
Living in the Moment

Dr. Landsverk makes navigating the medical and behavioral challenges for a loved one with dementia a bit easier to comprehend. The book explains what is happening, what is likely to happen, and how to do the right thing along the way. Recommended to family members who suspect their loved one might have dementia, essential to those with new diagnosis and no where to turn, validating and reassuring those who are already on the dementia journey with a loved one.

—**KJ Page**, Gerontology RN, ED, Joint Commission Nursing Center Policy

A valuable resource . . . [this] book is essential for understanding a confusing disease and navigating the medical, legal, and financial challenges for these vulnerable elders. Everyone needs this book.

—**Kim Schwarz**, CLPF, past president, Professional Fiduciary Association

Dr. Landsverk reveals the secrets to medical and personal care with people with dementia. Her insights tell you what to expect and how to fix things so people with dementia—and their loved ones—can live their best lives.

—**Marsha L. Keeffer**, CLPF, partner, Practical Heart Fiduciary Services

Dr Landsverk has shared a geriatrician's perspective to provide poignant yet practical insight with an exceptional level experience, to equip families for the journey ahead of them."

—**Nancy Schier Anzelmo** MSG, gerontologist, advisor to Alzheimer's Association and Dementia Action Alliance, founder Connected Horse

Provides lots of practical advice and information on a medical condition that remains a source of confusion for many families and doctors alike.

—**Carlos A. Camargo, Jr.**, MD, professor of emergency medicine, Harvard Medical School, professor of epidemiology, Harvard School of Public Health

Dr Landsverk's unique blend of intellectual competence and curiosity makes her an invaluable guide in finding a steady path forward with a diagnosis of a dementia. Her greatest interest is in identifying causes of distress and agitation to help elders better enjoy their lives. She works to treat unrecognized pain while improving the overall medication regimen.

—**Catherine Madison** MD, founding director, Ray Dolby Brain Health Center

Living
in the
Moment

**Overcoming Challenges
and Finding Moments of Joy in
Alzheimer's Disease and Other Dementias**

Elizabeth Landsverk, MD

with Heather Millar

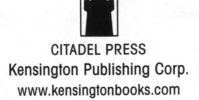

CITADEL PRESS
Kensington Publishing Corp.
www.kensingtonbooks.com

CITADEL PRESS BOOKS are published by

Kensington Publishing Corp.
119 West 40th Street
New York, NY 10018

PUBLISHER'S NOTE
This book is sold to readers with the understanding that while the publisher aims to inform, enlighten, and provide accurate general information regarding the subject matter covered, the publisher is not engaged in providing medical, psychological, financial, legal, or other professional services. If the reader needs or wants professional advice or assistance, the services of an appropriate professional should be sought. Case studies featured in this book are composites based on the author's years of practice and do not reflect the experiences of any individual person.

All Kensington titles, imprints, and distributed lines are available at special quantity discounts for bulk purchases for sales promotions, premiums, fund-raising, educational, or institutional use. Special book excerpts or customized printings can also be created to fit specific needs. For details, write or phone the office of the Kensington sales manager: Kensington Publishing Corp., 119 West 40th Street, New York, NY 10018, attn: Sales Department; phone 1-800-221-2647.

CITADEL PRESS and the Citadel logo are Reg. U.S. Pat. & TM Off.

ISBN-13: 978-0-8065-4177-8

First Citadel trade paperback printing: June 2022

10 9 8 7 6 5 4 3

Printed in the United States of America

Electronic edition:

ISBN-13: 978-0-8065-4178-5 (e-book)

*To my elders, who have taught me more
than medical school ever did.*

Living
in the
Moment

Introduction

NO AFFLICTION OF OLD AGE is more likely to be treated ineffectively than dementia. The onset of dementia is gradual, complicated, and subtle. Successfully addressing medical and behavioral needs requires finesse. Sadly, too often, the effort is unsuccessful.

I know about this firsthand. After graduating from the University of Virginia Medical School and completing a residency at Harvard, I worked as a primary care physician for seven years. One day, an older man came into my clinic complaining of chest pain. I tried to do an electrocardiogram to check his heart, but the man started hitting everyone within reach. He was out of control. I had to ask the staff members to take him away. It bothered me that I didn't know what to do.

The incident inspired me to do a fellowship in geriatrics—medicine for elders—at Mount Sinai Medical Center in New York City, one of the world's leading centers for research on treating people as they age. I focused on the mental health problems of old age. After finishing my specialty training in geriatrics, I became an assistant clinical professor at the University of California at San Francisco (UCSF). But while UCSF is one of the top ten medical research centers in the country, I found that academic medicine didn't suit me, that clinical care was my passion. I wanted to have more freedom to direct that care and more opportunity to teach the techniques that I had learned at Mount Sinai. Now I knew how to handle an elder who becomes uncontrollably violent at the prospect of a routine test. Even more important, I knew how to prevent the outburst in the first place.

I left UCSF fourteen years ago to form my own independent practice, ElderConsult Geriatric Medicine, specializing in house calls for older patients. I also served as medical director of a hospice providing end-of-life care. Education and outreach had become increasingly important to me. Doctors usually give talks to other doctors. I wanted to spread awareness in the community, to let lay people know about alternative ways of treating the mental health problems of old age, especially agitation, depression, and psychosis. I advocate using sedating drugs as little as possible. I emphasize behavior modification and lifestyle changes.

As a society, we tend to both undermedicate and overmedicate: giving too many tranquilizers to some patients while not addressing the pain or disruptive and irrational behavior of others. We are loath to take decision-making power from our elders, and we have imperfect tools to measure whether a person has "capacity"—the ability to run his or her own affairs.

The result is that many elders with early dementia suffer some kind of psychological, physical, or financial abuse. Then, when we do step in to manage our elders' lives, some of us take too much power, forgetting to allow them the freedom to choose what they eat, what they do, or whether they want to have a romantic partner.

Even more commonly, dementia treatment is nonexistent: Only one in five of those with symptoms of dementia have been diagnosed, according to testimony before the United States Senate.

Even when they're on the case, families, caregivers, and health professionals often find it difficult to assemble all the necessary information or resources to address the complete picture. Families may exhaust themselves—both physically and financially—caring for a demented relative, unaware of the many kinds of support available. Caregivers may grow frustrated, unaware that very simple adjustments to daily routines can sometimes make all the difference for a dementia patient.

At some time in our lives, almost all of us will

have to cope with these vexing problems. About 10 percent of people over age sixty-five suffer from failing brain function. After age eighty-five, that figure rises to approximately 50 percent, according to the Alzheimer's Association. Alzheimer's is the fifth-leading cause of death among people aged sixty-five and over, according to the organization's data. And while other major causes of death have decreased in recent years, the incidence of mortality due to Alzheimer's has risen 46 percent. This doesn't even take into account other causes of dementia, such as alcoholism, Parkinson's disease, or small strokes.

So perhaps it's not surprising that, again and again, I have met patients and families struggling to deal with the problems created by faltering mental function. And again and again, I have seen families completely overwhelmed—exhausted to the core, unsure where to go for information, and unable to untangle the intertwining medical, psychological, interpersonal, legal, and practical knots created by a loved one whose ability to think is failing.

It *is* possible for elders and their families to live fulfilling lives after a dementia diagnosis. I decided to write this book to give families a straightforward map and toolbox for the road ahead.

Before beginning any journey, you need to have some idea of where you are and how you got there. Then you can see where you're going. You can see your goals and what help you need to achieve them. Only then is it possible to survive, and even thrive, on this path. This book will give you what you need to do just that.

Anyone who's faced a medical or family crisis knows that during the first few months, the learning curve angles straight up. There is so much new information to absorb: new terms, new resources, new options, new questions, new processes. Dementia is *both* a medical crisis and a family crisis, and it strikes at the core of identity and relationships. That makes the affliction even more challenging.

A quick click around online or a browse through the local bookstore shows there's no shortage of books about aging and dementia. Some purport to hold the key that will lock out old age indefinitely. Hefty medical tomes outline advances in dementia research. Poignant memoirs bring on the tears. One man even chronicled his own descent into dementia. Giant overviews published by groups like the Alzheimer's Association or the . . . *for Dummies* book series cover just about everything you could ever want to know about the current state of dementia treatment. Several doctors have written books offering their point of view on the subject of aging and cognitive decline. All these works have their place, and I include a list of suggested titles and online resources for further reading at the end of this book.

However, I believe that in the midst of a crisis—in the first days, weeks, and months before and after a dementia diagnosis—families don't need emotive memoirs, encyclopedic medical explanations, or magical thinking. Since four out of five dementia patients live at home—and caring for these people is more than a full-time job—neither patients nor families have a lot of time for reading.

What's been missing is a concise, easy-to-digest overview of what you'll need to know for the months and years ahead. You want practical advice on just getting through the day. You need a smart reference for what to do *right now*, rather than spending hours flipping through pages and pages of details to identify the right one. That's what this guide does.

You also need to recognize that while dementia is a discrete medical condition, it affects the whole person and the whole family. Therefore, I believe that treatment should be holistic, with practical steps that take in all of life, from bank accounts to bathing and from depression to dental care.

Too often, when a dementia patient is suddenly violent or inappropriate or in danger of making a disastrous financial decision, various professionals discount these problems as "not part of dementia" or "something that must be endured" or "the elder's right to be foolish." Often, many of these problems can be solved by recognizing the signs of early dementia, by determining what care plan and team are needed, and by considering whether an adjustment of a medication is appropriate.

This means understanding what drives odd behaviors in dementia. It means working with the elder, not insisting that he or she faces the calendar that says it is a Wednesday in May. It means understanding what the world looks like to these elders and helping them with compassion and patience to navigate the bewildering world that this disease has made their reality. When all else fails, I strongly believe in using medications to treat the behavioral problems of dementia. This point of view remains controversial. But I have seen it work for patient after patient. Some of the families of these patients tell their stories in this book.

Families and patients also need reason for optimism. I fervently believe that dementia is a challenge that patients and families can meet with success. Dignity, grace—even joy—are still possible with the relevant information and an integrated plan.

All this requires preparation for the long haul. Dementia rarely runs its course in a year. Sometimes it may go on for a decade or more. Each situation has its own story, its own subtleties, and its own challenges. Dementia isn't as straightforward as a broken bone or a heart attack. Strange things can happen: A once-adoring spouse can turn violent and paranoid. A once-confident professional may suddenly suffer from crippling anxiety. A once-efficient executive may stop paying her bills or make loans without paperwork, giving away large amounts of money to unscrupulous family members and outright strangers.

Families need access to key facts about how the brain works and how different kinds of dementia lead to different behaviors. They need to know the early signs of dementia. They need to know how dementia is diagnosed and how it is treated. They need to understand how the world looks and feels to a dementia patient. They need practical advice on day-to-day living. They need to know the importance of putting their family's legal and financial house in order. They need to know the signs of elder abuse. They need to know how to find options for the support and care of both family and patient. They need to know how to judge whether a facility or a caregiver or a program is right for their loved one.

This book will cover these basics in short, easy-to-find, and easy-to-understand sections. It will outline the most common issues and resources. It will detail concrete steps to help you through the process in an integrated, holistic way. These are the things I would like every patient and family to know from Day One.

No book on such a vast topic can be all-inclusive. This guide shouldn't be considered as direct advice on medical matters, financial planning, or case management. What it can do is help you to ask the right questions of doctors, elder care lawyers, care managers, caregivers, physical therapists, occupational therapists, facility managers, and other professionals. It should give you the tools to determine the right solutions for your unique situation.

Let's get started!

CHAPTER ONE

First Things First

Y OU'RE READING THIS BOOK because someone you love has been diagnosed with dementia or you suspect that your loved one's forgetfulness or quirky behavior might be something more serious. You may be feeling confused, frustrated, hurt, or frightened. You may be aching with anxiety and grief as your relationship changes profoundly and permanently. The problem may feel so big that you're reluctant to look at it fully.

One of the most heartbreaking misconceptions I see in my practice is when families assume that a diagnosis of dementia means that life won't be worth living any longer. Nothing could be further from the truth. Life can still be rich. But this requires that we reconsider some of our assumptions and expectations about life and about dementia.

The biggest lie is that dementia means, "It's all over." Have hope. You can still enjoy good times together. A diagnosis of dementia doesn't mean the end of the world. Yes, a family's life changes when dementia enters in. Sometimes the shifts come dramatically: an elder will have a sudden health setback. Dad may go out for a drive and not be able to find his way back home. Mom may try to "escape" her assisted-living facility because she's convinced they are keeping her prisoner.

Yet, as we will see, these setbacks can be overcome. Life can continue to bring love, joy, and fulfillment. With the proper support and information, people with dementia can have engaging, enjoyable lives. I have helped thousands of families and patients find solutions to the challenges that make the elders miserable: untreated pain, medications causing agitation, lack of caregiving knowledge and strategies, or the needed level of care to live with joy or contentment, even as the decline progresses. Of course, the goal of this guide is to give you the ability to live with joy and contentment, too.

What it takes is proper care, support, and education. This book aims to begin that process.

You may wonder if you're overreacting. Does my loved one *really* have early dementia? How can I tell if there's really a problem?

First Signs

The earliest stages of dementia are the most difficult to identify and to deal with. Where is the line between eccentricity and dementia? Between normal forgetfulness and dementia? Between stubbornness and dementia? Between normal caution and demented paranoia?

Nearly every family I work with clearly remembers the confusion that set in when they first started to suspect that something was wrong with their elder loved one. Here are a few examples from relatives of my patients.

Ellen, about her mother-in-law: "She started leaving the oven on. She would forget to flush the toilet. She didn't remember if she had eaten or not."

Kelly, about her husband: "He had always been good with our finances, but he began to pay some bills late or he would forget to pay them at all. That wasn't like him."

Robert: "My father was only in his sixties when we noticed something was off. He was an attorney and always very organized. But he started to forget appointments, meetings, even my son's birthday. He forgot to take his medication. He forgot to do his taxes. His mail was piling up, but when I commented on this he got angry."

Brian, about his wife: "She started having problems at work. She had problems with her speech, stumbling over her words, forgetting some words completely. I started to notice that she'd use the same catch phrases over and over."

Forgetfulness is common. If these things happen once or twice, it may just be a mistake. But if you begin to notice a pattern, it may be time to check things out. If there are repeated financial lapses, you may need a trustworthy agent, like a fiduciary or a conservator, to manage their finances.

If you're comfortable discussing finances with your loved one, bring up what's causing your concern. If you see red-striped notices from the power company or the tax collector on the desk in your father's study, don't hesitate to talk to him about it. It's not snooping; it's protecting your loved one.

Often, elders are hesitant to turn over financial control to their adult children. In this situation, try to emphasize "the hassles of bills." At times it makes sense to have a third-party professional, especially when there is discord in the family. Explain that a professional fiduciary can take on that burden without taking control.

You may also notice behavioral and mood changes. In the early stages, an elder might appear reasonable most of the time. She might also, however, begin to spin suspicious tales, convincing the authorities that her husband is beating her or that a housekeeper is stealing or that a caregiver is climbing into bed with her. Of course, those stories should be checked out. But

it may well turn out that the husband simply pat-
ted her on the hand or that she misplaced her
pearls or that the caregiver must kneel on the
bed to help change her incontinence underwear.

The early stages of dementia may be the most
challenging for families. Without warning, their
loved one is acting strangely, cranky, and unpre-
dictable. It's difficult not to feel frustrated or
annoyed. It can feel as if the person is willfully
misbehaving, ruining the day on purpose.

The important thing to remember is that people
suffering from early dementia aren't trying to be
difficult. They can't help their perplexing behavior. They may not be consciously aware that they
have changed. Or they may be acutely aware of the
changes, and actively trying to hide them.

Home Test: Screening for Dementia

If you're not sure whether your loved one is having cognitive problems, try one or two of these
simple tests:

- Ask the person to draw a clock showing the time as ten minutes after eleven
  o'clock. (The trick is to put the long hand
  and short hand in the right places.)

- Ask him to name as many animals as he
  can in one minute. If he can list more than
  twenty animals, that's about normal.

- Can your loved one determine 25 percent of $22.50? If not, and that person does the finances, he or she needs evaluation. This is a simple calculation; if this is challenging, this person isn't able to address more complex financial decisions.

If your loved one has trouble with these and other areas of daily living, then it's time to go to a doctor—but not just any doctor.

Make an appointment with a geriatrician, a neurologist, or a physician recommended by the Alzheimer's Association. (General practitioners are fine for many medical issues, but they typically aren't accustomed to the subtle signs of early dementia.)

So, What Is Dementia?

Although dementia research has increased exponentially since the 1980s, there is still much about it that isn't yet understood. Here, briefly, is an overview of what we know.

First, let's be clear on what dementia isn't. It is not forgetting where your glasses are. It's not forgetting someone's name when you run into him at a party. It's not losing your train of thought when you're cooking dinner and trying to herd your children through their homework. These are normal lapses that affect all adults from time to time.

In casual conversation, the words *dementia* and *demented* may take on a variety of meanings, everything from "silly" and "goofy" to "hopelessly inept" or "crazy." In medicine, *dementia* has an exact definition with three key aspects.

1. A loss of short-term memory. It's not just forgetting names or not remembering what you were doing. The problems start when the patient *forgets* that he's forgotten, when his understanding of the past and of the future gets fuzzy. He doesn't just forget an appointment with the doctor; he forgets that he has been to the doctor and that the doctor has prescribed a change of directions for taking his blood thinners. He eats lunch and then can't remember doing so. When he asks for lunch, he's irritated to be told he just ate. This type of memory loss makes it difficult for the patient to properly evaluate situations.

2. Memory problems that interfere with the tasks of daily life. An assessment system used by medical professionals calls such tasks instrumental activities of daily living. They are simply what you need to be able to do to live independently as an adult: manage money, pay bills, shop for groceries, cook, and do the laundry, among other things. These are measures of so-called executive function and can be the first signs that something is wrong.

Someone who has reached this point will probably sound okay socially but not be able to function independently. That person has lost the ability to determine risk and to reason through abstract choices. He or she can be at risk from unscrupulous people who offer to take care of everything. With lower risk assessment skills, the elder is more likely to go along with plans that put personal finances at risk.

People with dementia lose control of their daily routines or the instrumental activities of daily living: missing appointments, leaving bills unpaid, not taking medications, not going out to get groceries, or not washing clothes. They become unable to manage routine tasks: balancing a checkbook, cleaning house, preparing a meal, or driving along familiar routes.

The ability to perform the activities of daily living, such as dressing, bathing, grooming, toileting, and, finally, even feeding oneself, declines as the disease progresses. The person often doesn't recognize the need for help.

3. Altered social behavior or personality. A shy person becomes promiscuous. An affectionate spouse becomes hostile. A trusting parent turns paranoid. Dementia makes it difficult to pick up on the social cues that we all rely on to interact with others.

Most people don't understand that dementia is extremely variable. It's not just forgetting; it takes many forms. That's because damage to different parts of the brain causes different sorts of behavior problems. Addressing behavioral problems is one of the central challenges of successfully managing dementia.

To understand how best to treat dementia, we need to understand how the brain works.

What Causes Dementia?

In the simplest terms, dementia occurs when the brain is damaged. This damage may stem from any number of causes: traumatic injury, small strokes, alcohol or drug abuse, or plaques (gummy lesions of protein that build up in the brain and block nerve connections). Whatever the cause, how the problem affects behavior depends on how extensive the damage is. It also depends on where the damage has occurred.

A Quick Map of the Brain

To understand your loved one's particular dementia, here's a basic outline of which brain structures do what.

- **The hippocampus,** with one lobe on each side of the brain, controls short-term memory. People with damage to this part of the brain may have a detailed memory of a football game thirty years ago but not something you told them in the last five minutes. They may ask the same questions over and over.

- **The temporal lobes,** one behind each temple, and the **frontal lobe,** behind the forehead, govern emotion, reasoning and social inhibition. People with damage in these areas may start acting inappropriately. They can be quick to anger over a little thing. They may burst into tears at the drop of a hat. They may have lost control of their impulses: They may eat to excess. They may grab someone they find attractive or misinterpret the actions of the young caregiver assisting with bathing as something they remember that had to do with their spouse and romance. They may decide on a whim to sell all of their possessions. This is where risk assessment and judgment reside, and they are often the first functions to go when dementia develops.

- **The parietal lobe**, at the upper back of the brain, helps with sequencing—that is, which things go first, second, and so on. People with damage to this area have trouble remembering how to put things in order. They struggle to work their way through a multistep process. They may put their underwear on after their pants. Or they may sit down to dinner but then not know what to do at the table.

- **The occipital lobe**, at the lower back of the brain, controls vision and balance. People with damage here have difficulty balancing, seeing, and reading. They may have trouble seeing in three dimensions. They may have a hard time sensing how far away something is or how deep a body of water is. They may perceive a black mat on the floor as a giant chasm. They may not eat because they can't determine where their food is, or they may not drink because they can't tell the color of the cup from the surrounding table. Oddly, their vision may test normal. They see objects clearly, but their brains aren't processing the information correctly. Glasses can't correct their vision problems because the trouble lies in the brain, not the eyes.

Dementia Comes in Many Forms

Dementia isn't just caused by Alzheimer's disease, though Alzheimer's is the most common and the best-known cause. There are many types of dementia, each with a different cause and subtle variations in symptoms. They each progress in very different ways.

- **Alzheimer's disease.** About 70 percent of those diagnosed with dementia suffer from Alzheimer's. The disease begins when amyloid proteins start to stick together, forming plaques between brain cells. These plaques appear to prevent the cells from signaling each other. Other proteins form tangles, or "fibrils," within brain cells. These tangles destroy the structure of nerve cells in the brain and eventually lead to their demise. As the patient loses more and more brain cells, his or her mental abilities begin to falter.

  People with Alzheimer's usually start to show symptoms and then begin a smooth, gradual decline until death. Once diagnosed, survival is typically four years for men and seven for women, though there have been cases as short as two years and as long as fifteen years.

In the beginning, the person becomes forgetful. He'll show personality changes, becoming more irritable, less empathetic, apathetic, or more anxious. Often, the loss of memory prompts those with Alzheimer's to become suspicious and paranoid. They lose the ability to perform routine tasks, like driving safely, cooking, using the telephone, or managing finances. Later in the course of the disease, they lose the ability to dress and to use the bathroom. In the terminal stage, they lose the capacity to eat and swallow.

- **Vascular dementia.** We've all learned to watch out for catastrophic strokes—blockages or bleeding in a significant blood vessel in the brain that can kill or severely damage a person's motor skills or mental abilities. But it's also very common for elders to have tiny "micro-strokes" involving blockage of smaller blood vessels, known as white matter ischemia.

The brain is made of gray matter, which are the nerve cells on the surface, and white matter, which are the nerve fibers found deeper in the brain that connect the nerve cells. White matter ischemia leads to little scars that damage the ability of the brain to work in various areas.

These white-matter ischemic changes are so common that doctors often consider them just a normal part of aging. Yet these strokes can cause very real changes in personality and mental function. Gradually, as more and more of these little strokes occur, parts of the brain begin to falter. This sort of dementia occurs in about 30 percent of people with dementia and may combine with Alzheimer's.

Vascular dementia randomly takes out bits and pieces of a person's ability to function, making it tricky to diagnose and to treat. A patient may still operate at a very high level in some areas but have debilitating "blind spots" in others. For instance, a patient may be able to play a complex card game like bridge yet be unable to remember to pay bills regularly.

A stepwise decline is the hallmark of this form of dementia. Vascular dementia progresses as a series of sudden decreases in function, such as abruptly losing the ability to sign one's name on a check or forgetting the name of the caregiver as the only sign of a stroke event. Some patients may be stable for months and decline in a stepwise fashion, slowly or quickly.

• **Alcoholic dementia.** Alcohol abuse causes brain deterioration that may eventually become dementia. Elders are much more sensitive to the effects of drinking, in part because they metabolize alcohol more slowly than younger people. Even one cocktail a day may render an older person at higher risk for dementia and decline. More than two drinks a day can result in chaos.

This sort of dementia can cause "dense" amnesia—a complete, or near-complete, loss of memory. In an alcoholic, other kinds of dementia, or any kind of mental illness, can't be diagnosed until the patient has been dry for six months. If the patient stops drinking, he or she can often regain some, but not all, lost mental function. Wernicke-Korsakoff syndrome is more common in alcoholic dementia and leads to confabulation (making stuff up), which might sound reasonable until you find out the real story. The biggest challenge is that once the brain damage leads to loss of judgment and disinhibition, there is no regulator on how much alcohol (or any other drug) is ingested until the person is managed in a controlled setting.

- **Lewy body dementia.** Abnormal protein deposits inside nerve cells, called Lewy bodies, are a common type of progressive dementia. These tau proteins scar brain function. The condition is also seen in Parkinson's disease, which is often marked by tremors, rigid muscles, and slowed movement.

One hallmark of this form of dementia is early-onset visual hallucinations—seeing everything from abstract shapes to departed loved ones. Disorders of REM sleep are also a hallmark. Most people are immobile when having dreams, but those with Lewy body dementia (LBD) often act out their dreams, kicking and hitting a bed partner. In addition to early onset visual hallucinations, LBD can also cause dramatic mood swings, from clear and sunny one day to delusional the next.

Unfortunately, medicines used to treat Parkinson's disease (drugs such as Sinemet (carbidopa, levodopa) that prompt the brain to produce dopamine (which regulates movement and mood) often worsen the paranoia, delusions, and hallucinations. As the disease progresses, the use of Sinemet may lead to more paranoia and delusions and a shorter period of improved movement. The doctor must attempt the delicate balance of enough Parkinson's disease medications to allow movement, but not so much that the person becomes paranoid, delusional, and angry. Progression of Parkinson's disease leads to stiffness, immobility, and finally loss of the ability to swallow.

- **Frontal dementia.** This dementia attacks the frontal lobes of the brain, the parts immediately behind the forehead that govern emotion, reasoning, social behavior, and impulse control. Patients with frontal dementia may seem to function normally. If asked by a doctor assessing their orientation, they can tell the date, time, and place. But they may also show incredibly inappropriate or unwise judgment. They may grope a caregiver who is trying to bathe them. They may give away tens of thousands of dollars they can't afford to lose to charities or swindlers. They may lose their speech or become obsessed with small details, to the exclusion of allowing daily care.

These patients run a high risk of financial harm. Because they can appear as socially normal, family and financial advisers may be slow to intervene in financial decisions. This leaves the field wide open for those who would take advantage.

"But I Don't Have Alzheimer's!"

Kevin, a retired architect, age eighty-five, has started shoplifting and bingeing on alcohol. Once shy, he has become hypersexual, groping women and sneaking into their rooms at his retirement community.

Kevin doesn't have Alzheimer's. He has frontal dementia, which causes damage to the frontal lobes of the brain, where we reason or make decisions. Such patients may be able to recognize neighbors and loved ones and can superficially sound okay socially, but they have serious lapses in judgment. They have lost the ability to determine risk and to reason about abstract choices. This kind of dementia usually results in serious impulse control problems. For Kevin, these changes have become so severe that he has problems managing his life. His behavior creates an uproar at his residence.

At a court hearing to consider placing him under conservatorship, Kevin stands up and says articulately, "I don't have Alzheimer's!" When most people think of dementia, they assume that an impaired person won't be able to recognize relatives or to carry on a conversation. But patients with frontal dementia can appear to be completely normal in brief social situations, like doctors' appointments (his doctor gave him a prescription of sildenafil [Viagra] recently upon request). This can mask acute deficits in abstract thinking such as the capacity to make complex financial or medical decisions.

The court declines to take action. Three or four months pass before Kevin gets appropriate legal protection. During that time, he is at risk of physical and financial abuse. His buddies may have figured out that he can't keep score for a round of golf, yet he retains control of his $600,000 retirement fund. If contacted by dishonest strangers or family members, he may give them large amounts of money for trivial services. It would be wonderful if this sort of abuse was uncommon, but in my experience, it happens every day.

- **Reversible dementia.** In rare cases, low levels of thyroid-stimulating hormone (TSH), vitamin B_{12}, or the nutrient folate can produce dementia-like symptoms. Correcting the deficiency can improve the condition. People who go for years without treatment for the venereal disease syphilis can also experience dementia. In these cases, treating the syphilis may improve the dementia, although it won't reverse the nerve damage. And, of course, the misuse of medications can make the elder look like he has dementia; a geriatrician can review the medications and indicate which medications are likely to cause problems for elders (see the Beers List). The most commonly misused medications are the anti-anxiety pills or sleeping pills: alprazolam (Xanax), lorazepam (Ativan), clonazepam (Klonopin), zolpidem (Ambien), or Tylenol PM (acetaminophen with diphenhydramine [Benadryl]). Anxiety pills must be tapered slowly, and the tapering often results in the elder looking more agitated from the withdrawal of the meds, not from the brain dysfunction itself.

Take a Deep Breath

All of this may sound very complicated and intim-idating. Think of this chapter as your basic road map, "Dementia 101." Go back to sections as you need to do so. And don't be afraid to ask more questions of the professionals who are helping you through this. With some information and context and perspective, I promise you that you and your family can navigate this challenging time.

CHAPTER TWO

Living in the Moment

FAMILIES NATURALLY GO THROUGH a grieving process when one of their members gets a dementia diagnosis and they all have to learn to accept that life has changed irrevocably. It's a challenge to let go of what you had. It can be frightening to face the uncertainty that the future holds.

Many of us have heard of the famous "Serenity Prayer," which is attributed to the twentieth-century American theologian, Reinhold Niebuhr, perhaps the most famous prayer written in modern times. The best known form may be a version popularized by Alcoholics Anonymous.

> *God, grant me the serenity to accept*
>
> *the things I cannot change,*
>
> *the courage to change the things I can,*
>
> *and the wisdom to know the difference.*

Stephanie Howard, a dear friend and dementia care director, has crafted what she calls "The Dementia Serenity Prayer." It goes like this:

> *What "was," was.* (In other words, you can't go back to the time before dementia entered your family life.)
>
> *What "is," is.* (Dementia is the new reality. It is what it is.)
>
> *There is nothing wrong with making the "is," the best "is" it ever was.* (The dementia can't be changed, but you can make life with dementia as good as it can be.)

Dementia is no one's fault. It affects people with little regard to social standing, habits, or general health. You can't change the fact of dementia. What you *can* change is how you react to it.

Learning to Live in the Moment

What's key to making life with dementia as good as it can be is the idea of "living in the moment." Try to understand that "now" is the primary reality of most dementia patients. Live in "the now" with them.

People with moderate to advanced dementia exist completely in the present. Memories that form the connective tissue of relationships are stripped away. This causes stress and grief for family members who are saddened that Mom doesn't remember their birthday or that Dad has forgotten what he once did for a living.

The loss can be very hard for people with dementia in the beginning, when they may know something is wrong but don't know exactly what it is. They may be told, "What do you expect? You're old!" The changes may leave the person distressed, depressed, and withdrawn—especially if no one will talk to them about their experiences. People at this stage commonly feel as if they're going crazy.

Mercifully, at some point, the person's stress decreases as the disease progresses. Bit by bit, as dementia gradually takes hold, the patient's awareness of his or her condition fades. When you feel upset or sad about your loved one's dementia, try to remind yourself that he or she very likely doesn't experience this same stress and grief. As they forget what dementia is, these elders simply don't agonize as their families do. They're not really worried about the future any longer, either. They're just enjoying whatever life is bringing in the current moment—sunshine, a meal, a cozy blanket. Imagine what a release that can be: they may still get angry or frightened, but they don't worry the way the rest of us do.

For families and caregivers, one of the best strategies is to try living in the moment as well, seeing the world of those with the disorder the way they see it. Try to understand that someone with dementia can't really change. If they can't change, then it's up to us to adjust our behavior, our attitudes. We can connect with and support them. We can help them to be as successful, as engaged with life, as independent as they can be, for as long as they can be.

The Story of a Sunny Afternoon

I'll never forget a warm, sunny afternoon in the garden of a dementia unit in San Jose, California. I sat there for thirty minutes. That's a long time for a doctor to be relaxing. I shared the sunlight with a woman resident, her daughter, and two other people under my care for dementia. Only two of us, the daughter and I, had full cognitive function.

Still, we had a delightful chat about the weather, food, and family memories. The conversation was not linear; it took interesting turns. The flowers were in bloom. We enjoyed the day, the sun, and the companionship. For a little while, those of us without dementia slowed down. We stopped worrying about plans, the next appointment, and the next thing on our "to do" list. The elders pulled us into their world. We became fully present in the moment, not worrying about yesterday or tomorrow. That afternoon was a blessing.

Life After Dementia Can Still Be Sweet

Dementia doesn't decrease enjoyment of the world and all it has to offer. In fact, patients may enjoy simple things even more than they did before the onset of their disease. For them, the stress of adult life—finances, worries about achievement, schedules—are melting away. What remains is "now": the smell of fresh-baked bread, the laugh of a grandchild, roses blooming outside a window, a game of golf or balloon volleyball.

A man and woman who both had early dementia fell in love and got married. Listening to music, holding hands, a nice dinner—simple pleasures like these make life worth living, even after a dementia diagnosis. I've worked with elders who, with help, still love to bake cookies or to take pictures. One couple went dancing regularly, well into the wife's dementia. They both loved it.

Unbelievable as it may seem now, when you're just getting used to the idea, the quality of your family's life could even improve with dementia.

The father who never had time for his family is now just happy to have someone to hold hands with and chat. One son reported that he had a much better relationship with his mother after she was diagnosed with dementia. "Mom was always nicer to company than she was to us children, and when she forgot who we were, she was much more pleasant to be with." His mother moved to a care facility where she was much better supported and engaged. She was happier than she had been when she was at home and when he was growing up.

Um, Why Was I Angry, Again?

One of my patients once was a successful attorney. Before alcoholic dementia and frontal dementia impaired her, she was a force of nature. She was used to being in charge and tolerated little disagreement from her family or employees. When her daughter moved across the country after college, then stayed away for family and professional reasons, the woman was angry and resentful for years.

Yet as the mother's dementia progressed, she began to mellow. She was still demanding, but she forgot many of the reasons she'd been angry with her daughter. When her daughter eventually returned home to help with her care, the two enjoyed a more placid relationship than they had in years.

The patient had aphasia, a loss of language functions, such as speaking, understanding what others say, and naming common objects, which is sometimes seen in Alzheimer's disease. But at Thanksgiving, she was able to tell her daughter, simply, that she was grateful that her child was home. She was living in the moment, not the past.

Though the daughter could not say so to her mother, she was thankful that the dementia had melted away her petty disagreements so that they could have that talk.

Expert Advice: Slow Down, Take Time to Understand

Tiffany Mikles has been working with elders in the San Francisco Bay Area as a certified senior adviser since 1988. While managing a dementia care unit, she saw that the families of her patients also needed help. She founded Dementia Care Coaching in 2006 to educate and support those families, and she also runs support groups.

Here are her thoughts on the early days after a dementia diagnosis.

"Often, it's the families that panic. They want to put things in place, get a caregiver in the house right away. They say, 'You can't go for a walk if you have Alzheimer's, you can't live alone if you have Alzheimer's.'

"I encourage families to step back. Someone you love has just been diagnosed with dementia, but tomorrow is going to be much the same as

today. It really is. People with early-stage dementia can often function pretty well.

"We do need a plan for the future, but we don't
need drastic measures right away. We need to
learn about the disease, to educate ourselves."

CHAPTER THREE

Why You Need to Act

WELL BEFORE DEMENTIA is finally diagnosed, families typically struggle for some time with the nagging feeling that something is wrong. Often, they delay action because they're unsure. Is Mom's sudden anger and anxiety just normal aging? Is Uncle Joe just discovering a new side of himself, or are his lewd comments something more serious? Dad forgot about that one appointment, but maybe it was just an honest mistake. Shouldn't old people be able to make their own decisions, even if they seem ill-advised?

Our society values individual independence. Families and courts thus rightly use caution when considering the possibility of limiting an adult's free will. Geriatric specialists seek to preserve as much as possible of their patients' freedom. Our preference is to help patients live their lives as they wish, in their own way.

Yet the reality of dementia cases runs counter to this understandable desire of individuals, courts, and doctors to preserve independence. A memory-impaired elder with complete independence can be a danger to himself and to others.

Afraid to Give Dementia a Name

Eleanor began to notice changes in her mother thirteen years before she was formally diagnosed with Alzheimer's disease. First, her mom had started to complain about driving. "It's too confusing! The other drivers are crazy!" She got lost on the way to a lunch appointment. Then she misplaced her jewelry and accused the housekeeper of stealing it. She became convinced that her husband, who was devoted to her, was cheating.

After several years of such incidents, Eleanor offered to take her mother to Puerto Rico. She hoped it would give her father a break. It was a disaster. Her mother didn't want to leave the hotel room. She saw people in the bushes. She was so unnerved by the new environment that she wouldn't go to sleep and wouldn't let her daughter sleep, either. It was worse than vacationing with a toddler.

When they got home, the daughter gently suggested that maybe Mom had some sort of dementia. Her father refused to discuss it. For a while, neither parent wanted to see their daughter. Though they eventually softened, both refused to talk about the mother's changed behavior and capabilities.

Years passed. The mother grew increasingly suspicious, refusing to let visitors or doctors into the house. The father's health started to suffer. Finally, the kids researched various dementia facilities. The father needed a knee replacement, and the kids used that as a pretext to get their dad out of the house.

They brought me in to evaluate their mother, who was ever more paranoid and irritable. I adjusted her medications so that she became calm enough to enter a dementia facility. (In my experience, antianxiety meds, such as lorazepam [Ativan] or alprazolam [Xanax], aren't a good choice to improve behavior long term in elders with dementia.) The kids finally convinced their father that Mom needed help. After years and years of being the 24/7 caregiver, the exhausted father relented. He had his surgery, and his health improved. His wife got better care in a dementia unit.

Actually recognizing that problems may have their roots in dementia is one of the most difficult things for families. Remember that the earlier a person is treated for dementia, the better the outcome. This is true not only in medical terms but also in terms of emotional, physical, and financial well-being.

Families who suspect that a loved one is suffering from dementia don't need to go from zero to sixty miles per hour in under a minute, but they do need to act as quickly as possible. Those who intervene early have the best chance of preserving their loved one's ability to function, the best chance of avoiding legal and financial troubles, the best chance of getting appropriate medical treatment, and the best chance of getting support so that the strain of caring for a demented relative doesn't overwhelm them and damage their own health. Comprehensive treatment includes identifying which medications to remove, the team needed for care, activities to enrich, treating pain, caring for needs, and determining which medications will help.

Dementia doesn't forgive delay or rationalization. You need to switch gears from being the agreeable spouse or the dutiful child to the advocate who prioritizes the need to safeguard the health and well-being of your loved one. The stakes are high. Left unrecognized or untreated, elders with failing brain function may suffer all kinds of disasters. The biggest mistake families make is ignoring their gut feelings. If you suspect there's a problem, don't explain it away. Check it out. Ask the neighbors what they observe. Make a report to Adult Protective Services. Research geriatricians in your area, and call for an appointment.

The Price of Inaction: Undue Influence

Elders with early dementia often get in trouble when someone tries to exert what's called "undue influence." In layman's terms, this means that someone is trying to take control over the elder's affairs and doesn't have their wishes or best interests at heart. All the abuser needs is an opportunity and a sense of entitlement. Unfortunately, con artists identify dementia much more efficiently than the rest of us.

It's easy to see how these situations arise. As dementia progresses, the older person feels lonely and increasingly lost. The kids may live far away. Or they may live nearby but be consumed with their own jobs, kids, and concerns. Someone—a driver, a housekeeper, a neighbor, a distant relative—steps into this void and becomes the elder's "fixer." Dad or Mom suddenly has a new best friend. Then the new friend starts asking for legal control (such as power of attorney; see chapter 12), money, or assets like cars and houses.

The House that Got Away

Cindy, an eighty-seven-year-old former school-teacher, needs money for car repairs. She decides to sell her house to a neighbor for *one-quarter* of its appraised value. Cindy's son, Liam, tries to intervene, but his mother says it's her decision, getting angry when her son tries to press the issue. Liam doesn't have power of attorney, nor is his name on the deed of his mother's home. With no legal recourse, he reluctantly decides to contact a lawyer to help get his mother declared incompetent. He doesn't want to take away his mother's independence, nor does he want to go against her wishes, but he feels he must protect her.

Cindy has a preliminary test of her mental function and gets a marginal score. Depending on how you look at it, she's on the low-functioning side of normal or the high-functioning side of dementia.

Although she can't remember the name of her neighbor, Cindy says she's sold him her house already. Her lawyer refuses to allow more in-depth neuropsychological testing and maintains Cindy is competent to handle her affairs.

Liam is advised to call Adult Protective

Services. The authorities conclude that the neighbor and the attorney seem above-board, and besides, Cindy's score on the preliminary test of mental function, the Mini-Mental State Examination (MMSE), is 25 points out of 30. A score of 24 or more is typically seen as suggesting normal cognition, but it is only a screening test. In this case, comprehensive neuropsychological testing would show the loss of judgment, resulting from decreased frontal lobe function, that leaves her unable to make reasoned decisions. Sadly, that detailed testing is not ordered, so Cindy can do what she wants. She sells the house to the neighbor for a ridiculously low price.

Not long after this, Cindy stops paying her bills, a common sign of early dementia. Her lawyer starts paying bills for her. When Cindy dies a year later, Liam discovers that he has been cut out of her will. In the changed will, all the assets go to the neighbor whose name Cindy couldn't even remember.

No doubt, Liam regrets not having discussions with his mother years earlier about her finances and preparing for a future when she might need some protection.

The Price of Inaction: Financial Abuse

The earliest days of dementia may be the most perilous to financial safety. An older person may appear to be just fine in a casual social setting and yet have seriously impaired judgment. There are legions of people ready to take advantage of the gap.

- Phone representatives from sweepstakes and lottery companies routinely call elders. It's not uncommon for an older person with faltering judgment to send tens of thousands of dollars to an overseas lottery.

- Elders who donate to one charity may be subjected to pleas from dozens of other nonprofits. People who've lost the ability to assess risk can have their assets drained by donations they can't afford.

- A contractor may accept payment for work, then never show up to complete it—or worse, come in and cause damage, then demand more money to fix the mess.

Unscrupulous caregivers may sweet-talk their employers into writing them checks for undocumented loans or giving them free access to their ATMs—may even suggest marriage. Forty percent of cases examined in a 1998 study by the

National Center on Elder Abuse involved some sort of financial abuse, amounting to 220,000 victims in a single year. About 30 percent of all crimes against elders involve financial exploitation, a higher percentage than the physical abuse that most families fear. In 2003, the U.S. Senate's Special Committee on Aging reported to Congress that more than three out of four cases of elder abuse go unreported. On that basis, it conservatively concluded that three million to five million seniors are taken to the cleaners annually. Financial abuse was estimated to have cost elders in America as much as $2.9 billion in 2009, according to a MetLife Mature Market Institute study.

Losing savings or a house to an unscrupulous person damages both the health and well-being of the patient. Over and over, I've seen patients make disastrous financial decisions that put them at risk.

- They forget to make mortgage or rent payments and suddenly find themselves in danger of foreclosure or eviction.

- They forget to pay the power bill or the phone bill and have their service cut off.

- They sell assets for a fraction of their true value. They may decide to give away their car just because someone asks.

- They take valuables like jewelry, which they had wanted to leave to relatives, and give them away to strangers.

- They relinquish their ability to make financial decisions by signing over power of attorney to a friend or a relative who wants to take advantage of them.

Granted, even people with normal brain function can fall victim to swindles. If the elder in your life is suffering from depression or grief over the loss of a loved one, is isolated or abuses alcohol or drugs, he or she is even more at risk. If your relative complains about money being missing or has signed confusing forms (such as a reverse mortgage) or can't find a treasured possession like a wedding ring or has suddenly arranged to have mail delivered to a different address—consider those red flags. Don't delay. Take action.

From Riches to Rags

Ronald was a successful doctor who retired in his midsixties, a wealthy man. Widowed in his seventies, he lived for five years with his son and his family, then moved across the country to be near one of his brothers.

Once there, Ronald hires a housekeeper who cooks his meals and cleans his house for the next ten years. Most of his family members live far away. Only his brother is nearby. Ronald has always managed his affairs and remains fiercely independent. So the family doesn't pay close attention.

As time goes on and Ronald becomes frail, the housekeeper gradually becomes his main connection to the outside world. Then he has a fall and is hospitalized. That's when his grandson gets a phone call.

The social worker tells the grandson, who lives on the opposite coast, that she doesn't think it's safe for Ronald to go home. The grandson flies across the country to find that his once well-to-do grandfather is nearly penniless.

After weeks of digging through records and organizing papers, the grandson pieces together what happened. His grandfather had given his ATM card to the housekeeper. The housekeeper had been withdrawing $300 to $400 every day for nearly a decade. The withdrawals far exceed her grandfather's living expenses. The housekeeper has also convinced her employer to trade his new Cadillac for her broken-down Honda, which now sits in the driveway of his home.

The grandson takes this evidence to the police. Yes, they tell him after looking over the paperwork, they believe the old man has been financially abused. Proving it, however, is another matter. It would be difficult to show that the withdrawals hadn't been made at his grandfather's request. Didn't he like to play the horses when he was younger? The housekeeper could just say she was withdrawing the money so he could gamble with it. Since his grandfather now suffers from dementia, there is no reliable way to ask him what happened. There is no case.

The older man is broke and not able to care for himself, so the grandson takes his grandfather to live with him. The family never sees the housekeeper again.

The lesson here is that, early on, the elder may look and sound completely fine, while having lost his or her "risk assessment" skills. It's imperative that you have conversations about finances with your loved ones early and regularly. If you suspect that your loved one has lost the capacity for making sound financial decisions, you will want to take action before it is too late.

In many cases, this loss in judgment can be picked up in neuropsychological testing. However, occasionally, the test isn't sensitive enough to pick up the loss of risk assessment correlated to damage near the temple at the front of the brain known as the temporal section of the frontal lobe. In this case, the Iowa Gambling Task can identify those who have lost their risk assessment ability but nothing else. The elder has lost the capacity for financial decisions if he or she can't assess risk.

The Price of Inaction: Physical Abuse

People with early-onset dementia are also far more likely to suffer physical abuse. Family members have to be on the lookout for this problem because the elders usually are in no state to explain or to set off the alarm. If they're in the early stages of the disease, they may not want to draw attention to their deficits, or they may fear being put away in a nursing home (as abusers often suggest). People with dementia may lack the organizational, motor, or verbal skills to draw attention to the fact that they're being mistreated. If you can't remember how to find out who might help, or even how to use a phone book, or what a public agency is or does, how can you alert the authorities? If you're having trouble forming sentences or remembering what happened yesterday, how can you tell a neighbor or a relative that you're being treated badly? If simple physical tasks, like opening doors, are getting difficult, how can you run away? Would you even know where to go?

At the same time that they may not be able to ask for help, elders with dementia are much more likely to do exasperating things that, over time, may drive even a loving caregiver to abusive behavior. Dementia tends to go hand in hand with behavioral problems: pacing, searching, repetitive questions, anger, confusion, paranoia, or extreme demands for attention. Caregivers or even relatives who don't understand the roots of this behavior may lose patience and lash out. They may not be aware that their actions may contribute to the patient's disturbing behavior.

Hard and fast numbers are difficult to come by. A study in the journal *Clinics in Geriatric Medicine* found a link between dementia and elder abuse. Also, about one in four elders in the general population are at risk of physical abuse, according to a review of forty-nine studies published in the journal *Age and Ageing*. Victims of elder abuse are three times more likely to die at an earlier age than those who aren't abused, according to the National Committee for the Prevention of Elder Abuse.

Abuse Develops One Step at a Time

Agnes married her high school sweetheart, Matthew. They had a generally happy marriage. As they aged, she promised never to put him "in one of those places."

But when Matthew developed progressive dementia, life got very hard for the couple. Matthew could no longer bathe himself; he walked unsteadily; he forgot to eat. He had delusions. He was often paranoid, especially toward the end of the day. Caring for Matthew became a trial.

Perhaps without realizing it, Agnes lost her patience. Now, she complains that she has to yell at her husband to get him to do things. When she helps him, she is often rough. She refuses to be realistic about what Matthew can do. She begins to discount his complaints. She doesn't do anything about the fact that he's lost fifteen pounds in three months. When he complains his arm is sore, she neglects to take him to the doctor. In the end, it turns out he has broken the arm in a fall.

Jane has asked her friend, Sue, not her son Tom to be her durable power of attorney (DPOA) and make decisions for her when she cannot for medical or financial issues. Jane has given him one of her three houses already. However, when she developed dementia and could not care for herself, and Sue was away for a month on business, Tom takes his mother to a lawyer and has her change the paperwork to give *him* durable power of attorney, and promptly cuts down caregiver hours and takes ownership of the other houses.

The son doesn't act responsibly at all. He leaves Jane alone in the house for hours on end. She loses even more weight. Because no one is making sure that her body is repositioned regularly in bed, Jane develops pressure sores. Finally, she passes out and is taken to the hospital. Doctors there find her thin, unwashed, covered in sores, and dehydrated.

The hospital calls Adult Protective Services. The agency investigates the son for elder abuse. Jane gets discharged to a nursing home.

Did Agnes and Tom set out to handle things so badly? Agnes probably not. Yet—mistake by mistake—her actions veered into abusive territory. Tom knew what he was doing and took advantage of his mother's vulnerability, when the DPOA was away.

Many family members are surprised to learn that abuse may come in the form of simple neglect.

Often, families struggle to take care of a failing relative at home. They may not understand the physical needs of someone confined to a wheelchair or to a bed. They may not know that a person who doesn't change position every two hours can suffer bedsores. They may not see that bedsores can lead to dangerous infections and an early death.

The Price of Inaction: Emotional Abuse

Every family has problems of one sort or another. Every family has dynamics that, in a perfect world, could be improved. But as an elder's abilities begin to fade, some of these relationships and interactions can gradually turn abusive. This is one reason why studies have shown that 90 percent of elder abuse comes at the hands of family members. Here are two such patient stories.

When Keeping a Promise Isn't Necessarily Best

I receive a call from the family of Clara, an eighty-five-year-old woman. She and her husband, Edgar, have been married for forty-six years. He sees it as his duty to care for her and not to "put her away."

Yet the husband clearly can't handle this obligation. He feels overwhelmed. Gradually, Edgar has become emotionally abusive. He yells at Clara for small mistakes like spilling a drink or soiling herself. She didn't *decide* to spill or to wet herself. She does these things because her abilities are impaired.

I listen to Edgar's story. He tells me of their whole life together. He explains the many sacrifices he's made to keep his spouse at home. "I can see you want to do the best thing for her," I tell him. "Many loving families," I assure him, "simply can't provide all the care that a frail elder with dementia needs."

After a long talk, Edgar agrees to let Clara be taken to the dementia wing of their assisted-living facility. That defuses what had become an emotionally abusive situation. Edgar can see his wife every afternoon and hold her hand. Clara can get the care and interaction that she needs.

A lot of elder abuse isn't really an event, but a process. It can just sneak up on a family. A situation often starts out mostly normal, then one thing changes. Then another. Gradually, what was once acceptable veers into the abnormal and abusive. Sometimes it's the very incremental nature of the change that makes it so difficult for other family members to decide whether to intervene.

When Does Leaning on Mom Become Abuse?

Patricia, age eighty-one, had always defined her life by being a caretaker. She took care of her husband, Bob, who was disabled from multiple sclerosis (MS), until his death. She prided herself on caring for her three children. She took special care of her youngest child, Connie, who had mental problems and had trouble supporting herself.

The other two children weren't sure when the dementia began. They kept asking each other, "Is Mom acting strange because she's stressed about our Connie? Or is it something more?"

Patricia helped Connie plan her wedding. Patricia helped again when the marriage foundered after two years. After the divorce, Patricia helped when Connie started to have serious mood problems. When Connie attempted suicide, Patricia offered to let her move in with her, in an assisted-living community. Connie was supposed to stay two months, only until she could get back on her feet.

Nine months go by, and Connie is still

living with her mother. One night, Patricia's eldest child, Carl, gets a phone call from the assisted-living facility. Patricia is lying on the floor of her apartment. She refuses to come out if Connie is present. She's afraid of her daughter, she says. Family and staff members arrive, and everyone calms down. Still, the other siblings are disturbed. Just who should be taking care of whom? Can their sister really still think it's their frail mother's duty to take care of her when she can barely take care of herself?

A week later, Patricia calls the facility manager. She says Connie has told her that she's taken some pills, that she's dying. It's all playing out with maximum guilt and drama.

At the apartment, the manager finds the elder woman frightened and her daughter raving and incoherent. Bit by bit, the situation has become intolerable. Connie is transferred to a mental health ward. Patricia moves to the dementia unit of her facility.

The Price of Inaction: Sexual Abuse

While it's not common, sexual abuse of elders does occur, mostly to women. It may not be clear-cut. Mom may complain that an orderly is trying to rape her when it turns out she was just having her wet underwear changed. But in other cases, abuse may be real. Don't panic or become paranoid, but also don't dismiss claims of sexual abuse out of hand.

Even for professionals, this is a challenging issue to evaluate. People with dementia often have delusions and make unfounded accusations. Perhaps the best way to guard against the possibility of sexual abuse is to do background checks and make sure that a vulnerable elder always has trusted supervision. Create a system of cross-checks to make sure that the patient-caregiver relationship doesn't veer into inappropriate territory.

The Price of Inaction: Deadly Accidents

Our society is reluctant to take away a person's car keys. In a country of subdivisions and far-flung suburbs, in a nation that enshrines personal freedom, losing permission to drive can seem like a death of sorts. It can spell social isolation, which in turn can lead to a host of other problems: withdrawal, substance abuse, depression, or neglected hygiene.

There is no denying that some elders pose a substantial risk when driving, according to the American Academy of Neurology. Yet several studies show that a considerable number of people with mild dementia—as many as three-quarters—can pass an on-the-road driving test.

There's no equivalent of an on-the-spot "drunk driving test" for patients with dementia. Some people suggest using the "grandchild test." If you don't think your loved one drives safely enough to be trusted in the car with your children, then you should take the keys away before that person can harm someone else's kids.

Studies have found that the assessment of caregivers is usually the most accurate predictor of trouble. If you think your loved one's driving is unsafe, don't back down. Make sure he or she has a driving test with your state's motor vehicles department or a driving coach. If the elder drives into a school bus, the consequences will be severe—physically, emotionally, and financially.

A Near Miss

Rusty, a retired airline pilot, had always prided himself on his independence—and his classic Jaguar sports car. But as he reached his late seventies, his eyesight and depth perception began to fail. Family members started to notice dings and scratches accumulating all over the car. He explained them away with a shrug.

"A lot of people seem to be bumping into me lately," Rusty said.

One evening, he met an old friend downtown for dinner. Driving home, at dusk, he hit another car. Partly frightened and partly in denial about the fender bender, Rusty didn't pull over to exchange information with the other driver. Rather than stop, he kept going home. Furious, the man driving the other car followed him several miles to his house. When Rusty got home, he barely slowed to activate the remote control to raise the garage door and drove straight inside. The man knocked and rang the doorbell. Rusty refused to answer the door.

Eventually, the other motorist called the police. Rusty refused to acknowledge the accident. The incident eventually found its way into small claims court. The matter dragged on until Rusty's dementia was diagnosed and a fiduciary, hired to handle his affairs, paid for the damage to the man's car.

Luckily, the experience so frightened Rusty that he didn't drive again. If he had, the damage could have been much, much worse.

The risk of accidents doesn't stop when elders get off the road. Simple household conveniences can become dangers. Seniors whose abilities are faltering are more likely to forget that appliances like space heaters have been left on or to neglect something simmering on the stove. Pots neglected over an open flame are one of the most common causes of fire in the homes of elders. At this stage, it's not safe for your loved one to live alone.

The Price of Inaction: Health Setbacks

One of the classic signs of early dementia is that patients start to neglect their hygiene. They may forget to bathe or to brush their teeth. They forget doctor and dentist appointments. They may lose track of their medications, taking them irregularly or not at all.

Forgetting something like a blood-pressure pill can have life-threatening consequences, such as increasing the risk of a stroke. Left unbrushed, teeth can decay, and that decay, left untreated, can turn into a dangerous abscess. Most people don't realize that dental infections can even be fatal. In rare cases, they can spread to the brain. Elders with tooth pain may avoid eating. Thinner and weaker, they can become too frail to survive the next hospitalization. Poor hygiene increases the risk of problems of all sorts and severities: skin ulcers, gum disease, yeast infections, festering wounds, and fungal infestations of the skin, fingernails, and toenails.

Delayed treatment also is associated with irreversible declines in day-to-day abilities. The earlier treatment begins, the more seniors can preserve what function they do have. While there is no cure for dementia, several interventions can slow the disease. Physical and social activities can fight the decline. Early diagnosis also makes it more likely that a medical team can find solutions to the complex lifestyle and behavior problems created by dementia.

CHAPTER FOUR

Defining the Goals of Care

WHEN CONFRONTED WITH AN INJURY or an illness in a loved one, it's human nature to respond, "Do everything! Whatever it takes!" Pulling out all the stops may make sense for a patient who's forty or sixty, even seventy. For someone who's eight-five or ninety-five, it may not.

The decision to take a less aggressive approach isn't necessarily based on age; rather, it's because the patient is frail. We do not advocate "slow medicine," but focused care for the goals of the elder. Those with dementia often feel under attack and become combative in hospital settings. To prevent elders from fighting the treatments or pulling out intravenous (IV) lines and monitors, they're often heavily sedated and restrained. This can lead to pressure ulcers, choking on food or phlegm, blood clots, delirium, and an earlier death. Aggressive treatment often means a worse outcome. This makes it important to figure out what doctors call the "goals of care." Simply put, this means defining why the patient is getting medical treatment in the first place: Is the goal a complete cure? Is it to make the patient as comfortable as possible? Is it to make it possible for the patient to stay at home? Is it to preserve function as long as possible? Ask yourself: What would your loved one want? Would he or she want to undergo the stresses of being in the hospital? To even be there? To be treated at all costs?

Consider a ninety-two-year-old woman with dementia who has become terrified of hospitals. She develops the flu—a condition that may demand hospitalization. If she is sent to a hospital instead of being treated at home, she won't understand what's happening to her.

A hospital is a very confusing and scary place for someone with dementia. Imagine being in that world of IV tubes, beeping heart and respiration monitors, blood draws, and uncomfortable procedures. Now imagine that you have no idea what's going on, why you're being put through all this. Frightened, the patient may become aggressive, fighting the hospital staff members—who will respond by tying the patient to the bed and sedating him or her.

Staying immobile in this way will put patients

at higher risk for bedsores, aspiration of food or water into the lungs, and blood clots. For every day that they spend in bed, they will lose 5 percent of muscle mass. Over five days that is a 25 percent muscle loss. Even if a patient sits up straight to eat (which isn't always the case) or lies flat after feeding, her increased confusion makes her more likely to suck in, or "aspirate," food into her airway. Aspiration can lead to pneumonia, and pneumonia is a major cause of death for elders. So, in such cases, the most aggressive treatment may actually hasten a patient's death.

An alternative is to have an evaluation done in the elder's home, a doctor or nurse practitioner house call, starting with antibiotics, if indicated for bacterial infection, and following up with a visiting nurse to make sure the elder is better. Care in familiar surroundings with familiar care-givers is much more comforting to those with dementia and fear of new environments.

One of the most disturbing things about dementia is the feeling that we are losing con-trol. We all have goals and hopes. We all like to feel that we have some power to decide things for ourselves. Over the course of a lifetime, we all develop a unique understanding of what's most important, what's most meaningful to our quality of life. This helps us to organize our lives.

As people grow older and less able to understand and cope, these goals and hopes inevitably shift. While a retired athlete may have wanted to remain healthy enough to play tennis, he later may become content with a daily walk. A woman who adamantly insisted on staying in her home may become so lonely and so infirm that moving to an assisted-living facility becomes a godsend, not a defeat.

It's important for families and patients to periodically review their goals and hopes with the medical and caregiving team. Remember that medical schools tend to emphasize curing disease. Most training programs provide only one month on geriatric medicine, and they devote even less time to the care of dementia. Few doctors spend more than a few days on special courses in end-of-life care. Psychologically, it's hard for most doctors to admit that they can't fix something. After all, most of them got into medicine because they wanted to triumph over problems, not learn to live with them.

Because of this reality in the medical culture, families need to be proactive. They need to ask the questions rather than wait for the medical team to do so. This process will be easier for everyone if patients, families, caregivers, and medical professionals can agree on the goals of care.

As you think about these goals, ask yourself:

What would my loved one really want? What can he or she expect to get out of treatment?

Often, the patient and the family might want different things. Many, many times I have had to face a son or daughter who wants to put the parent in a nursing home or wants a medical procedure that the parent doesn't want. I believe we should honor our elders' wishes rather than doing what makes *us* feel most comfortable. As much as possible, our feelings of fear and loss shouldn't get in the way of the patient's wishes. The eighty-five-year-old woman who lives alone and is falling frequently and can't remember she is falling and refuses help at home needs to have someone with a durable power of attorney or her chosen "decider" help determine what arrangements will let her be as independent as possible while living as safely as possible.

Every few months, or as changes occur, ask your family and your medical team:

- What are the priorities?
- What makes life worth living for my loved one? How can we best support that?
- How should the plan for care be structured to help achieve these goals?

Having a plan not only avoids many problems, it also actually enhances the quality of life. It helps everyone to cope, to respond, and to prepare for the future. The key is to agree on guidelines that honor the values of the person being cared for and then to make sure that everyone follows through.

The Hospital Is Not Always Best

Perry, an eighty-one-year-old man with moderate dementia, has become very agitated. He's taken to the hospital and is found to have a urinary blockage requiring a catheter.

When I first see him, he's been in the hospital for nearly four weeks and he's a mess: He has become delirious. The doctors give him general anesthesia and do a lumbar puncture to see if his spinal fluid might reveal the causes of his confusion. He needs a new catheter to drain his urine. The tube is held inside his bladder by a small balloon to prevent the catheter from slipping back down the narrow urethra. Upon waking, Perry becomes so agitated that he pulls out the catheter—balloon and all. That causes so much bleeding that he needs a transfusion.

Mittens are needed to restrain his hands so that he won't yank out any more tubes. His legs are restrained as well because he kicks. None of the hospital staff members

want to do more procedures on him. Perry
has developed a cough. His confusion and
restraints in bed put him at high risk for
aspirating food and developing pneumonia.
He needs an operation to help his bladder
drain, but the team have not planned to do
the procedure.

So what should we do with this man?
Should we keep him in the hospital, where
he's clearly miserable and at risk? Or should
we find a different solution?

I advise the family to move Perry from the
hospital to a facility specializing in dementia so that his condition can be stabilized.
The family hires a caregiver to stay with him
at all times. The facility's philosophy of care
discourages restraints, so they remove the
mittens (without asking his doctor). Perry
pulls out his catheter again. He bleeds heavily and is taken to another hospital. Luckily, a local urologist helps out and surgically
removes the blockage (using a procedure
called laser TURP). After five days of mittens
and restraints to allow him to heal, the catheter is removed. Perry, who had been immobilized for weeks in the hospital, is up and
dressed in street clothes and walking with
the aid of a walker. His delirium clears, and
he becomes more coherent than he's been

for more than a month. He grows content with the dementia facility.

Would we have reached this happy ending if Perry had stayed in the hospital? It's unclear. He had become very weak there, and complex surgical procedures in dementia patients often have poor outcomes. However, the alternative was to leave him sedated and tied in a bed—a miserable way to decline and die.

Some kinds of intervention should only be used to treat serious conditions, such as removing an infected gall bladder or pinning a broken hip. One of my patients, an eighty-seven-year-old man, had vascular dementia caused by impaired blood flow to the brain. After years of being aggressive, he had mellowed. He walked a little and enjoyed watching others at his residence. He was eating less and was on hospice care in preparation for death.

His wife grew concerned about a dime-sized skin growth on his cheek that wouldn't heal. A dermatologist said it should be removed in an operating room, with general anesthesia. I learned about the procedure after the fact, when I was notified that he was acting more confused and yelling at night. When I arrived, I could see that he had suffered a stroke. He died two weeks after the surgery. I would strongly advise that only procedures to address distressing medical situations, such as a hernia or a hip fracture, be treated. Follow-up mammograms, carotid ultrasounds, and small incidental findings should be avoided.

When it comes to some medical issues, we must think for our loved ones. Is the problem something that really affects quality of life? Is fixing it worth the risk?

When Less Is More

An older woman named Maribel has moderate dementia. All her life, she's avoided doctors and been skeptical of conventional medicine. One day, she feels a lump in her breast.

Both her family and her doctors need to consider: What's the most compassionate and sensible thing to do? Aggressive treatment of her cancer would most likely involve long and arduous IV chemotherapy and radiation—treatments she would never have trusted when she was competent and can't possibly understand now through the fog of dementia. If the chance of a cure is remote, would it make more sense to give Maribel a pill to shrink her tumor and leave her without serious side effects for her remaining time?

In her case, palliative care—that is, treating symptoms but not expecting a cure—was the kindest course of action. Her tumor responded, for a while, to an oral chemotherapy medication that did not have noticeable side effects. For Maribel, it meant more quality to her days without difficult invasive treatment.

In the context of modern medicine, setting goals and planning treatment for elders—those with dementia—becomes tremendously complicated and nuanced. Technology has grown so advanced that it's possible to keep people alive long after they've lost the capacity to enjoy even the most basic of life's pleasures. This doesn't contradict my argument that people with dementia can enjoy life. But for all of us, at some point, it's time to let go. No one wants an indefinite period of being hooked up to machines, immobilized, in bed, and unable to speak.

It's common for elders to develop complex constellations of ailments along with dementia. It may be possible to treat every disease, but it may not always be advisable. Sometimes the side effects of treatment can outweigh the benefits. Or perhaps a treatment, while effective for a short time, may be traumatic. A painful or uncomfortable scan, for instance, may yield more information about a patient, but what if the condition it reveals is untreatable? It's not always necessary to measure everything.

Goals of care should include consideration of risk. Sometimes a patient may desperately want to engage in an activity that's a little dangerous. Should we let patients take chances? It depends. Let's say an elder has a conservator who handles his business affairs. The man wants to invite friends to a party at the ballpark. He's always loved going to games there. The conservator says no, it's risky. But is it? How about box seats or a luxury suite, going early (of course, scoping out the bathroom situation), making it a party, and leaving after most fans have driven away? If the man has supervision and enough money and if this is what he wants, why not? Even if a patient has dementia, he often still knows what he likes.

Or let's say a woman with moderate dementia wants to have unproven, expensive, and experimental medical procedures. Might the doctor selling these treatments have undue influence over this patient? Does the woman have the capacity to weigh the risks and benefits? Can she make a rational decision? Past performance may offer a clue. Can she understand the risks and benefits of medical treatments such as treating diabetes or hypertension with the proper medications? If she can't understand why it's important to treat those common conditions, I would argue that she doesn't have capacity to choose risky, unproven treatments. Neuropsychological testing can offer a definitive verdict. It's likely she doesn't have the mental capacity to make this kind of decision—a complex problem with many pros and cons.

That said, families also need to beware of those hawking "miracle cures" for dementia, such as chelation therapy using heavy metals or dozens of supplements a day at a cost of thousands of dollars. There are no studies showing that these treatments have a beneficial effect. Slick sales pitches and long promotional videos do not replace evidence. Sadly, there are no cures for dementia. Think of it like emphysema or scarring of the lung. Dementia is scarring of the brain. If supplying needed Vitamin B_{12} or thyroid medication or correcting medication problems that can cause delirium does not improve thinking, it will not improve.

In addition, medical professionals must always be aware that medications affect elders more powerfully than younger adults. I've worked with many elders who were deemed to have "advanced dementia"—not eating well, not coherent, not functioning—who greatly improved in their ability to think, function, and enjoy life when their medications were corrected. Generally, elders shouldn't be on sleeping pills or anti-anxiety pills, which commonly cause more problems than they solve (see medications section).

There is also the concern that an elder with dementia won't get standard medical care for acute conditions simply because they have dementia or are just plain old. That is how a ninety-two-year-old woman with a damaged hip, who still works at the family business, was steered away from getting surgery by a doctor's recommendation not to attempt the repair because of her age. She did, ultimately, have her hip pinned and returned to working in the family business.

Another case involved an older man with acute pancreatitis who wasn't offered the standard evaluation of a magnetic resonance imaging (MRI) scan of the bile duct due to his mild dementia. Fortunately, he was taken to another hospital, where the MRI revealed that he probably had biliary duct cancer, which aided the family in making plans for care.

Or take, for instance, the ninety-four-year-old man whose lung x-ray showed a gray shadow—a sign of possible fluid buildup or infection—that didn't clear up after treatment with antibiotics. "Well," his doctor said, "we would not do anything anyway." However, the man became short of breath and needed emergency hospitalization for heart failure, which resolved quickly once he had the proper medication.

Elders need us to be their advocates. No one should be sent home without care or treatment for pain because they're demented and their symptoms aren't judged to have merit.

What Would You Do?

For a sense of the complexity involved in establishing goals of care, consider some of the questions that have presented themselves in my practice.

- A ninety-two-year-old man has dementia and emphysema that remains uncontrolled despite intensive treatment. He needs a carotid endarterectomy, a highly invasive operation to treat the narrowing of the main arteries supplying the brain and reduce the risk of a stroke. Does this make sense, given his age and already fragile health?

- A bedridden eighty-six-year-old man with alcoholic dementia also suffers from diabetes, liver disease, kidney failure, and many other ailments. He has a port, a device that provides a point of entry for medication, surgically implanted to be used for dialysis. But no one asks if he can realistically take on the challenge of traveling to a dialysis center every other day. He never goes to the dialysis center.

- Should a woman with a history of falls who feels compelled to constantly walk around her assisted-living facility be permitted to do so, even if it increases her risk of falls? Or might she be less stressed and more free to walk in a "board-and-care" home with a higher ratio of staff members to patients?

- A ninety-two-year-old man with advanced dementia is taken to the hospital with a prolonged seizure. A scan shows some shrinkage in his brain. This atrophy and the associated enlarged ventricles are more commonly associated with dementia in someone of his age and condition, but they also could be caused by normal pressure hydrocephalus (or too much fluid in the brain, causing dementia, incontinence, and poor gait). In someone two decades younger, standard procedure would call for a full neurological exam—brainwave EEG (electro-encephalogram), lumbar puncture, and a follow-up MRI requiring complete sedation. Or in this case, would simply providing an antiseizure medication to control the symptoms make more sense?

- An elder woman's dementia makes her incapable of understanding even simple health issues like why she needs to take her blood pressure medication. She develops anemia, which may be a sign of blood loss or colon cancer. She refuses to allow a blood sample. Should the anemia be investigated with a colonoscopy, the standard for a younger patient with full mental faculties? A colonoscopy will require uncomfortable bowel cleansing—drinking a little over four quarts of a powerful laxative, followed by constant diarrhea. Should she go through this? There's only a one-in-a-thousand chance that her bowel may be perforated. If there's a problem found, it will require surgery. Her family has made it clear that they don't want that. Given her level of dementia and the one to two years of life probably remaining, would it make more sense to just give her iron tablets to reduce the discomfort of her fatigue from the anemia?

Dr. Louise Walters has done studies showing that screening for cancer makes sense only if the older individual has a prognosis of living an additional ten years or more. So a sixty-eight-year-old man with somewhat advanced dementia is unlikely to benefit from screening for prostate cancer. A seventy-two-year-old woman in good health may be a good candidate for breast-cancer screening, but one with dementia at that age may not.

Remember that dementia is a terminal illness. It is not survivable. If your brain—command central—doesn't work correctly, the body may send signals of pneumonia or a heart attack or even constipation, but the brain can't interpret those signals or communicate the problem in order to get help. With modern medicine, few adults die from pneumonia. In those with moderately advanced dementia, the risk of dying from pneumonia is 25 percent with treatment.

If those with dementia have other serious conditions, such as emphysema or congestive heart failure, these conditions may get better with hospitalization. Yet every time such elders enter the hospital, they're at a heightened risk of dying— from infections that live in the hospital, from medications, from the restraints used to keep confused patients in bed that can lead to bedsores, from falls, from sedation, from blood clots, and from aspiration of fluid into the lungs. With issues such as these, it can make more sense to localize the elder's problem, to fix the condition that causes discomfort or distress, and to keep the elder at home as much as possible.

Each family and each health-care team will answer these questions in different ways, depending on the situation, the medical prognosis, and the wishes of the elder and the family. The point is that it's important to discuss goals before there's a crisis.

Questions to Ask

When considering how to care for a person with dementia, be sure to consider the bigger picture. Hopefully, some of these issues will have been discussed before your loved one becomes severely impaired. In the best case, you'll have outlined these plans in documents such as an advanced directive, a living will, or a medical power of attorney. (See chapter 12 for more on these legal issues.)

Yet many, if not most, families don't have the luxury of time to plan ahead. It's important for all concerned parties to sit and discuss your loved one's care. The point is to ask what your loved one would want, not what you would want. Here are some questions to talk over.

- How has your loved one lived life? What are his or her general values and beliefs? Did your loved one prepare any advance health-care directives? If not, what statements did your loved make about growing older?

- Before your loved one got sick, what was most important in his or her life? What do you think is most important now? What activities are most enjoyable now?

- Given what you know about your family's wishes and your loved one's wishes and condition, what are your central goals? Prolonging life? Preserving quality of life? Avoiding suffering? Maintaining function? Maintaining as much independence as possible?

- How has your loved one coped with medical procedures, such as drawing blood? What's his or her attitude toward more invasive life-extending measures, such as intubation? Resuscitation? The likelihood of returning to a prior functional state after cardiac resuscitation for elders over age seventy with chronic medical problems is less than 1 percent. If an elder does survive resuscitation, he or she will likely have much worse brain damage.

- What are *your* expectations? Although no one can say for sure, how do you expect your loved one's dementia to progress?

What are your fears for your loved one? What do you hope to avoid? What are you afraid might happen? What are your fears for yourself?

• If your loved one can't speak for himself or herself, whose guidance would he or she trust? What would he or she want done?

• Do you know everything you need to know to clearly understand your loved one's situation? Are there things about your loved one's condition that you don't understand or that need to be clarified?

• How are decisions to be made and information to be handled? This can be thorny because of federal privacy law. It's important to identify all the important players in the family and how they will share information, who has the authority to make decisions (durable power of attorney), which family members have strong views, and how differences will be resolved. This is especially the case with blended families (e.g., a new spouse, children from a previous marriage). Early meetings with mediators to clarify medical and financial plans are crucial.

• If your loved one has several goals, how would you rank them in order of importance? Which goals are for the benefit of your loved one? Which goals are for the benefit of other family members?

- Does your health-care team feel that your family's goals are medically realistic? Does your family clearly understand the prognosis for the diseases that affect your loved one?

- If a cure isn't an achievable goal, can the disease be stabilized?

- If it's not possible to cure all the patient's diseases, which conditions can most effectively be treated?

- What is the balance between the risks of the treatment and the effectiveness of the care?

When All Is Not Clear

Herbert has fairly severe dementia. He can't remember much of what happened yesterday. "You never come see me!" he tells his daughter, even when his daughter has visited the day before.

Herbert has painful nerve damage that needs strong medications such as methadone and Lyrica (pregabalin). He is bedridden and can't move, and he suffers from bedsores.

Three times in a year, complications have required the insertion of a flexible plastic tube into his windpipe, a procedure known as intubation, to help him breathe. This is an invasive, uncomfortable procedure that people with dementia may not understand. Such elders often fight to remove the tube.

In Herbert's case, each time, the doctors stopped his pain medications because narcotics can depress breathing. However, abrupt withdrawal (decreasing more than one-half of the current dose every few days) leads to excruciating pain that increases a person's blood pressure and heart rate. Herbert can't speak because of the tube, so he can't communicate his misery to the doctors.

After the last intubation, one daughter suggests that Herbert be admitted to a hospice for end-of-life care. Other family members are unsure. Some worry about making such a decision. However, since Herbert doesn't remember the previous day, he doesn't remember the pain of intubation or the pain that ensues when his medications are discontinued.

The family continues to talk to Herbert.

Gradually, everyone agrees that he doesn't know the consequences of his earlier choice to take extraordinary measures to sustain his life—what he called "everything done." Not putting Herbert into hospice care, they decide, would increase the risk he would die with tubes everywhere and in serious pain. They all know that Herbert wouldn't want that.

Herbert goes to a hospice, where he is much happier. He gets more attention. His pain is better controlled. His bedsores get better with more attention and repositioning, which are now possible because the pain has decreased.

- When should the focus shift from trying to cure someone to using interventions aimed at relieving suffering? How does your family feel about this? What does the doctor say?

- Does your doctor take pain management seriously? Some medical professionals believe that if a patient doesn't complain about pain, there is no pain. Unfortunately, patients with dementia may not be able to identify the source of their distress. When those with dementia hurt, they may act out or they may become withdrawn. It is a mistake to treat agitation from pain (such as distressing arthritis or muscular/skeletal pain) with a sedative like lorazepam (Ativan), rather than with pain-control measures such as long-acting Tylenol (acetaminophen); physical therapy; a TENs unit (electrical stimulation); topical application of diclofenac sodium (Voltaren), gabapentin (Neurontin), or pregabalin (Lyrica) and, in more severe cases, Norco, a combination of acetaminophen and hydrocodone (often only one-half tab two or three times a day); or low-dose methadone for severe neuropathic pain not responsive to other treatments. As has been widely documented, long term use of medications like ibuprofen (Motrin) or naproxen (Naprosyn, Aleve) should be avoided since they are associated with increased risk of heart attack, stroke, gastrointestinal (GI) bleeding, or kidney failure. Of course, there is the caveat of treating narcotic-associated constipation: observe and adjust the dose for sedation or increased risk of falling. The concern about escalating narcotic doses for elders with dementia is minimal if the elder is not managing his or her own medication and the caregiver is educated and reliable. Most people with dementia do not know what medications they are on and are not drug seeking. Treating pain effectively should be the first step in person-centered care. There is a school of thought that all chronic pain is mostly emotional. However, for elders with bone-on-bone arthritis, spinal stenosis or even a hip fracture, it is the quality of life that counts. Remember that those with dementia who undergo surgery have an increased risk of complications and further brain damage. Hundreds of elders who had reported severe pain in the past, do much better with less psych medication when their pains are treated with the needed pain medicine.

- Does your doctor see the bigger picture? A person with moderate to advanced dementia may have two to six years to live or might die at any time. Will your doctor take that into account when suggesting a treatment plan? For a woman of seventy-five with advanced dementia, there's little point in screening for cancer since she has a prognosis from her dementia of less than ten years of life.

- What if the patient doesn't understand what the surgery is for or why he or she is in the hospital? What if the disease may not cause a major problem? The misery of an inflamed gall bladder or enlarged prostate demands immediate intervention. But that's different from removing a skin cancer to prevent future medical complications.

- Is it more sensible to focus on day-to-day measures, such as flu vaccines and regular dental check-ups, that have a direct effect on the patient's quality of life?

- What living situation for your loved one will best balance financial constraints, medical and emotional needs, and the wishes of the patient?

- How can the elder's distress be minimized?

- How can the patient get the most out of every day?

As you ask these questions, remember that the answers shouldn't be what *you* would wish for yourself and your family. The goal is to find answers that conform to what your loved one would want, given his or her past actions and current situation.

Also, remember to take into account that what your loved one enjoys at the current stage may be different from what he or she preferred in the past. A love of opera, for instance, may now be satisfied with sing-alongs. A gregarious person may be happy with family visits three times a week and balloon volleyball on the other days. Of course, each person should be given the choices to participate in the activities of that person's preference. Remember, an elder will not likely have the stamina for prolonged events as in years past.

Sometimes the Hospital Hurts More than Helps

Roger has moderately advanced dementia. He also suffers from moderately severe anxiety. Sometimes he grows so anxious that he becomes aggressive and delusional. He takes lorazepam (Ativan), a strong tranquilizer, to manage his distress.

His wife takes him to a local memory clinic affiliated with a prominent academic medical center. The clinic refers Roger to the hospital for tests that might explain his dementia: an MRI scan, a lumbar puncture, and a carotid ultrasound. The hospital stops his drugs abruptly to avoid interfering with the tests.

Confused and agitated without his usual medicines, Roger inhales food into his lungs and contracts pneumonia. The doctors insert a catheter to drain his bladder. Roger goes home after a week.

At home, though, Roger becomes feverish. A urine test shows that he's gotten a drug-resistant infection from the catheter inserted at the hospital. He had entered the hospital in reasonably good physical health, but now, he is a very sick man. All this might have been avoided if he'd only had the tests that would affect his current care (for a person with advanced dementia, results from a lumbar puncture and carotid ultrasounds for dementia evaluation are not likely to change treatment) and not been admitted to the hospital but had a head CAT scan (computerized axial tomography) as an outpatient.

Finding the Solution that Works Best for Your Loved One

There is not a one-size-fits-all approach to any of these questions. You need to decide what works best for your loved one and his or her unique situation.

Kris, an eighty-two-year-old woman with dementia, feels a compulsion to walk. She sometimes walks so much that she doesn't eat, even though she is living in a facility that specializes in people with her condition and might be expected to keep a closer eye on her. Medications calm her somewhat, but she still feels an overpowering need to walk.

Kris becomes weaker and starts having falls. The family faces a difficult choice: Do they keep her confined and safe, or do they allow her to keep walking, which she enjoys and finds comforting?

I've seen this kind of falling-lady drama played out in several ways.

In one case, the doctor straps the patient to a chair. The restraints make her even more agitated, so he sedates her. She declines quickly.

In another case, the woman's family knows that her mobility is very important to her. Some families can afford twenty-four-hour, one-on-one care, but many cannot. After prolonged discussions with her dementia care facility, the family members sign a waiver stating that they understand that her walking puts her at risk of falls, but that they want her free to continue. They also say they don't want strong sedating medications used. The team works hard to assist her in walking the halls, keeps her in the community room where she can be supervised, and leaves her alone when she is in a low bed that she cannot get up and walk from without assistance. Despite the team efforts, she falls occasionally until she gradually becomes too weak to walk and spends her time in a wheelchair cruising around the community.

In yet another case, a woman needs to walk but can't be supervised in the large nursing facility where she lives. Her family decides to move her to a board-and-care home run by a nurse. In this smaller context, the woman can be more closely supervised. She can walk without being restrained, but with closer supervision.

Each family has to decide what is right for them, always guided by what they think their loved one would want.

CHAPTER FIVE

Getting a Formal Diagnosis

GETTING A DEMENTIA DIAGNOSIS brings on a host of feelings: fear, grief, confusion, anger, despair. For some people, it's a confirmation of what has been suspected. For others, there is a wave of denial. Everyone has a lot of questions.

Certified senior adviser Tiffany Mikles counsels families who are coping with dementia and also moderates related classes and support groups.

She says, "Often, families are nervous about discussing dementia openly with the person who has just been diagnosed. They're unsure what to say or whether they should say anything.

"Here's a simple strategy that works for me: I ask early-stage patients, 'Are you sad about this?'

"That really encompasses the whole thing. People are thinking, 'I thought I was going to have this lovely retirement; I thought I was going to travel. Now, I have to wear this bracelet that says I have dementia. I had no idea my spouse was going to have to care for me.'

"When I bring out that word *sad*, it all unfolds. None of us want to talk about that, but it's the only gift I can offer. I can't change the dementia. I can't make it better. But I can acknowledge that you're feeling sad. You're grieving the loss of the life you anticipated. So let's talk about that."

Each patient, and each family, is different. Some people want to be completely open about a dementia diagnosis. Others want to be completely private. And, of course, there are many compass points between those poles.

One family I treated wanted to be open, but they found themselves exhausted from endlessly having to make explanations. They came up with an ingenious solution: They prepared a two-page fact sheet describing the diagnosis, what friends and family might expect, how they could help, and where to find more information. Each time they had to tell someone new, they gave them the handout. They felt that the more friends and family members understood, the more they could talk with them.

How Is Dementia Diagnosed?

Diagnosing dementia is always problematic. The symptoms are varied, may appear in combination with ones from other diseases, and involve a part of the body—the brain—that is imperfectly understood. In the case of Alzheimer's, besides experimental scans, only an autopsy that finds evidence of the telltale plaques and tangles between nerve cells can yield a definitive diagnosis.

Sometimes early cognitive loss may be identified as depression. Depression and dementia can look very similar. People suffering from either affliction may eat and sleep too much or too little. They may feel hopeless. They may suffer from a loss of energy. They can't motivate themselves.

Remember that losses—the end of a career, the death of a spouse—and lost abilities can trigger depression. It's understandable when someone who experiences his or her powers slipping away feels low. If you can't do the things you used to do, mood naturally suffers. A hallmark of clinical depression is that the elder doesn't enjoy the things he or she used to enjoy. Most often, treating depression will improve the person's ability to function.

When dementia is suspected, a physician will order tests. Here are a few of the most common.

- **CAT scan/CT Scan.** Computerized axial tomography or computerized tomography combines several x-ray images taken from different angles to create a cross-sectional or three-dimensional picture of internal structures. The images demonstrate strokes, tumors, and bleeds that may also affect brain function.

- **MRI scan.** This type of scan, magnetic resonance imaging, shows more detailed architecture of the brain. However, in most cases, if a CT didn't show a tumor or another structural problem, the extra sensitivity of the MRI is unlikely to change the course of treatment for all but those with early dementia. In addition, people with dementia and those with claustrophobia may be more hesitant to spend fifteen minutes or so in the tight confines of the MRI tube rather five minutes in the open CT apparatus.

- **The Mini-Mental State Examination.** The MMSE questionnaire gives a quick snapshot of cognitive capacity. It evaluates orientation, asking patients to name the day, date, month, year, and season. It asks them to pinpoint address, city, county, state, and, when appropriate, building floor. It tests attention and recall: Patients must identify three objects and then recall them after doing another task, such as spelling *world* backward. It asks patients to repeat a phrase, to read a set of instructions, and then to complete a three-step task. It asks patients to copy shapes and then to write a sentence.

The MMSE test has 30 points and a score of 24 or more is generally said to be normal. However, it's a crude test. It does nothing to test judgment or abstract reasoning. I have seen patients score a 30 on the MMSE yet still lack the tools necessary to manage money or run a household. Thus, it often does not detect cases of early dementia.

- **The Montreal Cognitive Assessment.** The MoCA is a screen that tests a bit more for abstract reasoning, such as drawing trails between numbers and letters that are arranged in a pattern. It also is available in different languages, which is important because being tested in their primary language helps elders to do their best. However, this test is not definitive. If an elder has functional decline but aces the test, more testing is needed.

- **Neuropsychology evaluation.** Standardized neuropsychological tests investigate the relationships between various brain behaviors, which doctors call "cognitive domains." These include attention and concentration, language, memory, visual/spatial judgment, and "executive functioning," which is the ability to plan, initiate, and follow through on tasks.

The process usually involves interviews and a variety of written tests and other activities. The extent and expense of this testing vary widely. A healthy adult might be tested for four hours or more. At times several shorter sessions are required for an accurate assessment. If an elder becomes fatigued or irritable, the tests should be suspended for another day. Of course, it is important to have the person's medications assessed and adjusted to make sure the function we see is from the person's brain itself and is not affected by the use of alprazolam (Xanax), acetaminophen with Benadryl (Tylenol PM), oxybutynin (Ditropan), or levetiracetam (Keppra), which can all adversely affect cognitive function and behavior.

A neuropsychological exam isn't generally needed in cases of advanced dementia. It's more useful in earlier cases, when there's a question of diagnosis after a preliminary screen, such as the MMSE or the MoCA. Neuropsychological tests may help parse out the relationship between depression, personality disorders, and dementia that may be causing the lack of judgment.

If a family has concerns, it's a good idea to test before big problems exist. It can also be useful if an elder exhibits subtle changes and family members are concerned.

- **PET scan.** Positron emission tomography is a scan using a tracer that binds to the amyloid that deposits in the brain of people with Alzheimer's disease to more clearly identify plaque lesions in the brain. It is suggestive of disease, but there are also cases in which a person's function is better than the scan would predict, so this test should still be considered experimental.

- **Lumbar puncture.** A lumbar puncture, or spinal tap, can be used to sample the spinal fluid for levels of the amyloid proteins that cause plaques in the brain. In this case, a *low* amyloid level is concerning because it could mean more of the protein is being deposited in the brain, raising the risk of dementia.

In addition, rarely, a condition called normal pressure hydrocephalus causes a rise in the pressure of a fluid found in the brain and spine. The fluid then backs up in spaces of the midbrain known as ventricles. The ventricles enlarge, putting pressure on brain tissues and compressing them. This can result in rapid loss of bladder and bowel control, trouble walking, and dementia. Those symptoms are relieved by withdrawing spinal fluid and decreasing the pressure.

More common, however, is the *shrinking* of the brain (atrophy) from dementia, which can appear on a CT scan like the result of increased pressure in the ventricles.

- **Blood tests.** Low levels of vitamin B_{12}, folate, or thyroid-stimulating hormone (TSH) can cause dementia-like symptoms. Supplementing the missing compound can improve mental function but not often reverse the dementia. Simple blood tests can rule this out.

- **Syphilis test.** Syphilis, the sexually transmitted disease, can also cause symptoms that mimic dementia. This kind of dementia doesn't usually appear until the syphilis is quite advanced. In these cases, treating the syphilis probably won't significantly reverse the cognitive loss.

CHAPTER SIX

Treatment:
The Standard of Care

A S OF NOW, THERE IS NO CURE for dementia. However, there are basic lifestyle changes and medications that can slow the disease and improve a patient's ability to function. Physicians call this basic approach to a disease the "standard of care." What follows are the most important points about the standard of care for dementia treatment. Not everything in this chapter will apply to every elder, but it gives patients and their families an idea of how medical professionals and caregivers try to manage the disease. To be clear, there are no supplements, treatments, or medications that cure dementia. If someone tells you differently, that is just one of the many salespeople looking to sell the hope of a cure that does not exist.

Healthy Body, Healthier Brain

Studies suggest that about half of dementia cases could be prevented by healthy lifestyle choices. As with most diseases, it's difficult to overstate the importance of diet, sleep, exercise, and social interaction. Sometimes, in a minority of patients, inherited genes increase the risk of dementia, and while we can't pick our families, we can decide how to eat and live.

The key is to make lifestyle changes that will help preserve as many abilities as possible. All elders function better when they stay active, both physically and mentally. With dementia, as with so many other things, it's a "use it or lose it" world. Controlling blood sugar, cholesterol, blood pressure, and general fitness can make a huge difference. It can decrease the risk of developing dementia. It can also slow the progress of the disease once it develops.

Monitor Blood Sugar

As we all know, it's easy to gain weight as we age. As a nation, we have put on too many pounds. More than two-thirds of Americans are overweight or obese. Weight that is carried around the waist creates an increased risk of dementia, cardiac disease, and diabetes.

The major sign of diabetes is high levels of

blood sugar, which is called glucose. The sugar level rises because the body's cells don't respond properly to insulin, the hormone necessary to process the glucose that our cells need for energy. In the type 1 form of the disease, which usually strikes younger people, blood sugar rises because the body doesn't produce insulin in the first place.

Diabetes in older people is most commonly type 2 or non-insulin-dependent diabetes—when insulin can't be used properly, often due to an increase in weight. When glucose can't be processed by the cells, it remains in the bloodstream, increasing blood sugar levels.

Diabetes leads to many problems: kidney failure, heart attacks, strokes, infections, and blindness. It increases the risk of dementia through small strokes and probably through other inflammatory processes that we don't completely understand.

Controlling blood sugar is key to managing dementia. Changing lifestyle and eating habits, rather than taking glucose-lowering medications, is the best way to do this. If blood sugar levels rise too high, often over 200 milligrams per deciliter (mg/dL), there's a risk of infection. People with dementia react far more severely to infections. A simple bladder infection can result in agitation, even delirium. Nor is it good if blood sugar levels dip too low, because that has been shown to make dementia worse. It may also cause seizures. Recent studies show that using insulin more aggressively in patients with type 2 diabetes results in a higher death rate. Also, having lower blood glucose levels did not decrease the risk of death. Rather, improving lifestyle through increased exercise, weight loss, and a plant-based diet decreased glucose levels and the risk of heart attack, stroke, and dementia, too.

When treating younger adults, physicians try to keep blood sugar levels in a narrow range, say 80 to 120 mg/dL. But controlling glucose too tightly can cause problems for elders, increasing the risk of strokes and other cardiovascular events. So for a frail older person, a moderate range should be the goal: say 100 to 200 mg/dL.

Blood sugar levels need to be watched closely if a person isn't eating or drinking well. A variety of problems—a reaction to a new medication, a heart attack, constipation, or a bladder infection—may also dampen enthusiasm for food.

If an elder has reduced appetite, is forgetting to eat or unable to eat, or has kidney problems, doctors usually reduce any diabetes medication by half. Otherwise, blood sugar levels may dip too low.

Control Cholesterol

Almost everyone knows that it's important to control "bad" cholesterol, or LDL, the soft kind of cholesterol that can clump and form block-ages in arteries. Cholesterol control decreases the risk of heart disease and strokes that can lead to more rapid progression of dementia. Daily exercise and a high-fiber, plant-based diet with limited sugar and processed food is the simplest and most cost-effective way to control cholesterol. But diet alone may not work for all patients.

A whole family of drugs called statins has been developed to help lower cholesterol lev-els. Statins work by blocking a substance that is essential for cholesterol to be produced. These compounds include simvastatin (Zocor), pravastatin (Pravachol), atorvastatin (Lipitor), and lovastatin (Mevacor). In clinical trials, these drugs have reduced heart disease and the risk of stroke after two years.

However, the body's reaction to statins changes as it ages. While statins may dramatically decrease heart disease risk for a younger person, the effects may not be as great for those over age eighty-five. Side effects of statins can include liver inflammation, muscle weakness, and pain. They may diminish appetite and function.

These side effects may eventually outweigh the benefits, especially if the patient is becom-ing weaker and eating less. For a person with advanced dementia and a prognosis of two to three years of life left, the benefits of statins decrease and the burden of side effects increase.

Easy on the Blood Pressure

As with cholesterol, it's nearly impossible to avoid messages about the value of keeping blood pressure low. The target range for most elders is 130 over 80. The first figure, the higher of the two numbers, means the pressure in the arteries when the heart beats; the second measures the pressure in the arteries between heartbeats. The first number is called systolic; the second number is called diastolic.

As people age and become frail, they stop eating as much, and this can lead to a dip in blood pressure. Systolic blood pressure (the top number) below 100 can lead to strokes or dizziness and falls.

Scientists have found a connection between increased strokes and a significant decrease in blood pressure. That means that, as we age, blood pressure medication may need to be reduced so that the blood pressure doesn't get too low. Be sure to discuss this with your doctor. Elders with congestive heart failure or liver or kidney failure may have different needs.

Eat Well

With dementia, what you put into your body is hugely important. It's a matter of balance: Too much salt can lead to high blood pressure, kidney disease, and strokes. Too little salt can bring on low blood pressure, body chemistry imbalances, malaise, and even seizures when levels get very low. Too much sugar and too many calories lead to diabetes and that disease's complications. Too few calories or not enough protein leads to weight loss, weakness, and frailty.

Eating a healthy, balanced diet is a simple way of promoting cardiovascular health and avoiding the heart attacks and strokes that can lead to dementia.

The regimen depends on the situation. If a person has elevated blood pressure or glucose levels, which increase the risks of heart attacks, strokes, and dementia, then it makes sense to decrease the excess saturated fats found in fried food, butter, fatty meats, and cold cuts. Unsaturated fats—from nuts, olive oil, canola oil, or avocado oil—are much better choices. Limit servings of protein to the size of a deck of cards and restrict simple carbohydrates like cake and bagels. Replace them with a plant-based diet full of fruits, vegetables, nut butters, and whole grains. Some people claim that grains cause dementia, but there is no evidence for this. No studies anywhere link grains to decreased brain function. Rather, the fiber in whole grains helps delay the rise of glucose in the body. This, in turn, decreases insulin spikes, which decrease appetite, blood sugar, and cancer risk. One percent of the population has Celiac disease and should avoid wheat, rye, barley and any other gluten containing grains to decrease inflammation in the gut. Remember that alcohol is like a sugar and is not helpful for brain function. Older adults may enjoy a drink occasionally. But for those with dementia, it is best to avoid alcohol completely. Alcohol use in later years is definitely toxic to the brain.

Elders who have become too thin need direction from a doctor and a dietician about the best way to increase protein and calories and achieve a healthier weight. Sometimes something as simple as a milkshake or soy protein-powder shake once or twice a day can do the trick.

The Ice Cream Diet

A healthy diet may mean green, leafy vegetables and chicken or fish for a younger person. For an older person with dementia who won't eat anything, a good diet may mean ice cream and a liquid diet supplement like Ensure or Boost. Focus on what will give the person pleasure, as well as on fluids, calories, and protein.

One woman with moderate dementia, Becky, just stopped eating. Her sister and brother wanted to have her admitted to the hospital. They wanted to have many tests done. But over the preceding eight months, Becky had refused to agree to a colonoscopy to investigate her anemia. Eventually, the family realized that if she wouldn't consent to biopsies and other invasive tests, then she would never consent to surgery. Finally, she did agree to a barium test to help doctors see the outline of her esophagus and stomach.

It turned out that Becky had presbyesophagus, or changes in the mechanism of swallowing, which meant her esophagus could no longer move solid food down to her stomach properly. Yet she did just fine eating only ice cream and Ensure and taking iron for anemia. She lived for a year this way before dying peacefully at her residence facility.

Keep Moving

Just as we have "use it or lose it" brains, we also have "use it or lose it" bodies. Exercise and a plant-based diet are the only treatments that studies show will decrease the risk of dementia or the progression of dementia. If exercise were a pill, it would be more expensive than Viagra. The more we move, the healthier we are. This goes for people with dementia as well. Exercise helps lower glucose, cholesterol, and blood pressure.

Supplements do not help to decrease the risk of death created by too much glucose. Improving lifestyle with a plant-based diet and exercise is the only effective response. Movement and activity is the only way to delay frailty, the term used in medicine for the loss of muscle strength and bone density that comes with age. Staying active decreases restlessness, promotes deep sleep, improves appetite, and helps maintain normal bowel movements. Because regular exercise increases the fluids in the joints, movement also decreases arthritis pain. Daily exercise has been shown to slow the progression of Parkinson's disease. Even a gentle activity, such as yoga or the slow, deliberate movements of Chinese shadow boxing or tai chi, has been shown to improve balance, decrease the risk of falls, increase strength, and positively impact mood.

If your loved one hasn't been active for some time, consult a physical therapist before starting a new exercise routine. This will help to avoid injury.

Most people with dementia will face periods when they must be inactive, such as during hospital stays for illness or injury. Every day an elder stays in bed, he or she will lose 5 percent of their muscle mass. That means that a ten-day stay in the hospital may cause a 50 percent decline in physical strength. In such cases, it's important to consult a physical therapist as soon as possible, at the start of a hospital admission.

Those who are most frail get the most benefit from physical therapy. An evaluation by a physician and a physical therapist will help to identify the safest way to be more active.

Home Test: How Fit Are You?

Often, older individuals and their families will overestimate what elders can do. When it comes to fitness, safety is paramount. A serious fall can set off a precipitous decline.

One of the most serious injuries from elders falling is a broken hip. A quick way to judge if people are at risk is to ask them to get up from a chair of moderate height, such as a dining room chair, without using their hands.

If they succeed, it's a sign that their upper leg strength is pretty good and they have less risk of fall and fracture. Those who can't get up from a chair without using their hands are at higher risk; physical therapy should be the first step to increase strength.

A Medication Primer

The most direct drug treatments for dementia seek to improve the supply of key brain chemicals or to improve cardiovascular health that will avoid the mini-strokes that can cause dementia. In caring for your loved one, it's a good idea to know a little about the most common medications prescribed for their treatment. Use this section as a reference. When doctors suggest certain medications, you can look them up here.

Each drug has benefits and risks. The following information is general and should never be used to pick medications without the primary medical provider determining what is right for a particular elder.

Cholinesterase Inhibitors

The most targeted drug for dementia is **donepezil (Aricept)**. It increases the concentration of the chemical acetylcholine, which is important for the processes of memory, thinking, and reasoning. The drug is referred to as an acetylcholinesterase inhibitor or an anti-cholinesterase because it prevents the enzyme cholinesterase from breaking down acetylcholine.

Studies show that this class of drugs may

modestly help slow the rate of decline and possibly keep the nursing home at bay for an extra six months. However, the drugs only help 10 to 30 percent of those with dementia, and it's impossible to know which individuals will benefit. Therefore, it's common to give these medicines to all patients with declining brain function.

Donepezil is not a cure-all. While it is perhaps the best studied of the dementia drugs, its use remains controversial. It is expensive and the benefits are modest. There is no clear proof that the drug alters the course or the progression of Alzheimer's. Studies show better effects in brain function for Parkinson's disease, but this medication is not appropriate for frontal dementia.

In addition, donepezil's side effects may be uncomfortable. These include insomnia, nausea, loss of appetite, diarrhea, and decreased blood pressure and heart rate. Occasionally, the drug causes behavioral problems, such as agitation or sedation. Still, donepezil is certainly worth trying, particularly a low dose in the morning. This medication should not be used in the treatment of frontal dementia.

Several similar drugs also affect choline uptake.

- **Rivastigmine (Exelon).** This drug may be delivered by a skin patch as well as a pill.

The patch may be especially useful for patients who suffer from stomach upset or loss of appetite. However, with patch delivery method, the drug may make balance worse. With medications, there are always tradeoffs.

- **Galantamine (Razadyne).** This drug has side effects similar to donepezil. Some patients suffer from agitated behavior. Others don't seem to enjoy any benefit.

Glutamate Drugs

Memantine (Namenda) affects how nerves absorb glutamate, another chemical that helps brain cells communicate. It's thought that in Alzheimer's patients, brain cells take in too much glutamate. This may lead to an overstimulated state that makes the cells die.

Some studies have shown that prescribing donepezil and memantine together may be more effective than donepezil alone. Memantine's use is controversial because it may leave patients oversedated or confused. I have had some patients benefit from this medicine. For many, however, this medicine doesn't make a difference or they're too far down the road for drugs to be helpful. There is no reason to buy the more expensive combination pill Namzaric (Donepizil/ memantine) if your insurance does not cover it.

Drugs that Decrease Stroke Risk

"Baby aspirin" (81 milligram) thins the blood and decreases the likelihood of strokes that contribute to vascular dementia. It is more cost-effective than any other medication. The biggest side effect of thinning the blood is that it increases the risk of bleeding—mostly in the stomach, but sometimes from injury as well, such as bleeding in the brain after a fall. This risk can be decreased with a proton pump inhibitor (PPI) like **omeprazole** (**Prilosec**), which is the most common and inexpensive. However, the PPI can lead to low vitamin B_{12} absorption as well as increased risk of antibiotic-associated diarrhea that is caused by the bacterium Clostridioides difficile (C Diff).

Baby aspirin generally shouldn't be used with **clopidogrel** (**Plavix**), a drug used to prevent blood clots. If an elder has a stent keeping a heart artery open, aspirin or clopidogrel with other blood thinners may be prescribed, but the benefit may not be greater than the falls risk in a person with dementia who has lost safety awareness and is impulsive. Those with risks of falls are more likely to fall and bleed in their head than have a cardiac event.

Aggrenox, a combination of aspirin and **dipyridamole (Persantine),** may be used for those with peripheral vascular disease.

Clopidogrel (Plavix) also thins the blood and is more effective for stroke reduction than aspirin. However, some medications used to protect the stomach, such as omeprazole, **esomeprazole (Nexium),** and **pantoprazole (Protonix)** may prevent the clopidogrel from working. Further, clopidogrel may cause excessive bleeding. There's no quick way to reverse this side effect.

Warfarin (Coumadin) reduces the amount of vitamin K, which is needed for the formation of blood clots. Today, it is less frequently used to reduce the occurrence of strokes. This is particularly true with those who have atrial fibrillation of the heart, blood vessel narrowing, or replaced heart valves. This drug can be affected by the patient's diet and alcohol use. Those taking it need to be monitored closely for blood thinness and a significant bleeding risk.

Apixaban (Eliquis) is a common blood thinner replacing Coumadin and the need for blood testing, for atrial fibrillation or treating deep vein thromboses. The down side is that there is not an "antidote"; it must wear off, it cannot be reversed and should not be combined with other blood thinners.

Alcohol and pain medications such as aspirin,

ibuprofen (**Advil**), and **naproxen** (**Naprosyn, Aleve**) may thin the blood even more when used with other blood thinners. If a patient has already become confused and falls frequently, the risk of increased bleeding is probably more of a danger than the risk of stroke. For those on warfarin, vitamin K is an issue. Too many green leafy vegetables or a multivitamin with vitamin K will reverse the blood-thinning effect and increase the risk of stroke.

Medicines that May Make Dementia Worse

Most drugs specifically developed to improve dementia seek to increase the levels of choline, a chemical that brain cells need to communicate with each other. Yet several common medicines are anticholinergic. That is, they block the neurotransmitter choline. These drugs can make dementia worse, resulting in more confusion and agitation. They can also cause dry mouth, constipation, and difficulties urinating.

The more common include:

- **Diphenhydramine** (**Benadryl**) is an antihistamine found in cough syrups and over-the-counter allergy and sleeping pills such as Tylenol PM (in combination with acetaminophen). **Guaifenesin** (**Mucinex**), a common ingredient in cough medicines, is a better choice. It thins the mucus without worsening confusion or keeping the person from coughing.

- Bladder pills such as **tolterodine (Detrol)**, **oxybutynin (Ditropan)**, **trospium (Sanctura)**, or **solifenacin (Vesicare)** may be used to treat spasms that cause loss of urinary control. However, their side effects may include confusion and agitation. Cutting caffeine and diuretics may be a better alternative. Some urologists use "off-label" nortriptyline (**Pamelor**) at a low dose to decrease bladder spasms.

- **Atropine (Lomotil) or hyoscyamine (NuLev)** may be used to reduce respiratory secretions toward the end of life. Hospices often turn to them to relieve the distress of family members hearing the "death rattle," a sound that patients near death often make when saliva collects in the back of the throat. These drugs decrease the secretions, and hence, the noise.

However, if these drugs are used when the person is still conscious, they may cause severe confusion. Atropine may also be used for glaucoma in an eye drop form, which also can cause confusion.

- **Amitriptyline (Elavil)** is a medicine used in the past to treat depression and now prescribed to treat neuropathy and irritable bowel conditions. A related drug, **Pamelor**, can be helpful and cause less confusion.

- **Diphenoxylate combined with atropine (Lomotil)**, which is used to relieve diarrhea, may be okay if administered only once or twice. But if used regularly, its anticholinergic effects may cause problems for dementia patients.

- **Steroids**, medicines commonly used to reduce inflammation of various sorts, may also pose a problem for a person with dementia, causing confusion, insomnia, and agitation (also called delirium in medical contexts).

  When the steroid **prednisone** is used to treat emphysema and other lung diseases, its use should be reduced fairly quickly. Studies report little benefit to continuing this drug for more than two weeks.

- **Levetiracetam (Keppra)** is a newer antiseizure medication that is more reliable to use than the commonly prescribed phenytoin (Dilantin). However, it has been found to be associated with paranoia and aggression as well as sedation in some people.

In chapter 8, I will discuss the use of medications to treat behavioral symptoms of dementia. This is a controversial subject because there's a sense that it's an insoluble problem with little evidence for effective treatment. In fact, a recent review of many studies of medications for behavioral symptoms concluded that nothing works. And some commonly prescribed drugs—certain antipsychotics and tranquilizers used to control behavior—may actually make a patient more agitated or less socially inhibited. However, I have seen many cases where medications have helped. It's all a matter of weighing the risks and the benefits and looking for solutions to improve the patient's quality of life. I will discuss this fully later in the book.

CHAPTER SEVEN

Dementia and Behavioral Problems

MOST BEHAVIORAL PROBLEMS ARISE from unmet needs. The patient is lashing out because he or she's hungry or misunderstood or bored. Behavior is communication, but it may be expressed because of the brain damage that complicates his or her understanding of the world. Dementia does more than just render people forgetful and confused. It also commonly makes people anxious, paranoid, angry, and depressed. Dementia may make elders delusional. They may think that the president is coming to get them in Air Force One or that the hospital has been taken over by Nazis or any number of fantasies. Families seldom realize how common truly disturbing emotional and psychological challenges are among dementia patients.

An elder can be receiving excellent, compassionate care and still exhibit extreme behavior:

calling out endlessly, crawling out of windows, trying to hit caregivers.

I always advocate simple, practical solutions first. "The storm cannot hurt the sky" is a saying worth remembering when you have a family member struggling with dementia. If he or she is acting out but that behavior doesn't create any practical problems (such as danger to the caregiver or the elder), then it may be best to try to just live with it. Absorb the behavior as the sky absorbs the storm. The person with dementia is more likely to reflect back the attitudes he or she is receiving. Be open and patient and smile; it goes a long way.

Never lecture an elder with dementia for "bad behavior." He or she won't understand and will reflect back your irritation. Communicate in a pleasant manner. Talk at a pace the elder can process—only one idea or task at a time—and wait for the elder to understand and then respond.

Many behaviors shouldn't be treated with medication. Rather, people with cognitive decline should be engaged in activities they find rewarding. They should be free of pain. Their family members and their caregivers must slow down enough to understand the world *as the elder sees it*. Only then can they help the patient navigate the parts that don't make sense, with love and empathy.

Sometimes, unfortunately, these measures don't work. And the behavior challenges may become so severe that they interfere with the medical and day-to-day care of these loved ones. The elder refuses crucial diabetes medications, thinking he or she is being poisoned. Even with a gentle approach, a warm bathroom, and towels to cover the elder, a caregiver can't give a bath to someone who keeps trying to strike out. If a patient needs help eating but tries to bite the caregivers, how can they keep the patient fed?

I use a test similar to one used by addiction counselors: If the behavior is interfering with the elder's ability to live his or her life, then it's something worth dealing with. In these more severe cases, I advocate the cautious use of medications. Often, treating pain adequately and with a more gentle medication, such as long-acting acetaminophen (Tylenol) and low-dose gabapentin (Neurontin), which is an anecdotal treatment to decrease pain or anxiety, or more gentle selective serotonin reuptake inhibitors (SSRIs) such as sertraline (Zoloft), escitalopram (Lexapro), or mirtazipine (Remeron) may decrease the elder's distress and the behaviors that failed to respond to other measures.

If those treatments don't work or the elder is a danger to himself or herself or others or is inconsolably distressed by delusions and paranoia, I use more complicated psychoactive medications. At times mood stabilizers like valproic acid (Depakote) or antipsychotics are needed to calm these serious symptoms.

This remains controversial, but working with thousands of families with distressed loved ones has proven that it often may be the most effective and most compassionate approach. Yes, these medicines can have serious side effects. Antipsychotic medications increase the risk of stroke by 2 percent and raise the risk of sudden death by 1 percent. The numbers may seem small, but they're not trivial. I have seen a few patients (out of hundreds) have a stroke soon after the medication was given. The distress the elder is experiencing must outweigh this serious risk.

Such drugs shouldn't be used for general restlessness, such as patients who repeatedly say, "I want to go home, I want to go home." They shouldn't be used for the convenience of the caregiver, just to help the elder sleep, or to replace engaging activities. However, they should be used when the behavior is endangering the elder or others, when the behavior prevents needed personal care despite the best behavioral approaches, or when unrelenting distressing delusional thoughts cause daily misery.

Most importantly, these medications are *not* to be used to sedate an elder into submission.

If a patient is sedated, the cause needs to be evaluated. The sedating medications must be held back and any medical issues treated, only restarting the medication at a lower dose if serious symptoms persist. This elder should be examined every one to two months and the medications tapered when the person is doing well. The medical condition changes frequently as the disease progresses. We must adjust the treatment frequently, as well.

The list of troubling behaviors that elders with dementia exhibit is long indeed. They may forget or refuse to eat, or they may eat the same meal again and again because they can't remember having eaten. They may refuse to bathe or change their clothes. In their mind, they've just done those things and how dare someone suggest they can't handle such simple tasks? Because they can no longer distinguish help from a swindle, they're at risk. They may be easily influenced by traveling salespeople or by charity fundraisers. Caregivers, and even people they meet on the street, may take advantage.

The Most Common Behavioral Symptoms

Agitation

Agitation is one of the most common challenges in dementia care. In my practice, I find that it often underlies other behavior challenges. It develops at some point in a majority of elders as the disease progresses, and it may pop up when you least expect it.

Agitation can include being easily upset, anxious, or restless, pacing, irritability, yelling, threatening, repeating words and phrases, asking the same questions over and over.

In the early days, people with dementia may be frustrated by their inability to navigate the world they knew. Their capacity to plan and get things done, known as executive function, is off, and they get angry at small things. They can't understand why others are trying to pay their bills or take their car away; they've never had problems with that before. Those with vascular dementia caused by small strokes are more commonly engaged and present in the moment, but they cannot remember what happened before and may therefore think someone is stealing from them. They may misperceive the purpose of help or safety measures (such as having a caregiver in the home).

Toward the end, when they no longer seek to make sense of things, elders may get agitated because they can't communicate what they want or what's bothering them. Some don't want to be touched, even for needed toilet care to prevent skin ulcers. Caregivers who understand dementia patients are crucial to help people with dementia communicate their needs and wishes, and this alone can calm many situations. Sometimes the best medicine is to provide enjoyable diversions and simple pleasures, like ice cream, music, and an upbeat attitude.

Paranoia

As some with dementia feel their mental acuity begin to slip, they begin to doubt themselves. They forget where they put things—not just glasses but also the car they parked at the mall. However, others have no self-awareness and think it is all the fault of (fill in the blank; usually the person who has given up his or her life to help the elder—the spouse, the adult child, etc.). It's not unusual for a person with dementia to become paranoid about money or the car; of course those are two things that loved ones often do try to take away when they perceive that the elder doesn't have the capacity to handle them.

Dementia patients may become angry with visitors and doctors. They count as an enemy anyone who is telling them there is a problem or keeping them from what they think they should be doing. They may become convinced that their food is poisoned. They may come to believe that their spouse is cheating on them or that their spouse is an imposter.

Wandering

If the world seems unfamiliar to people with dementia, it makes sense that some will go looking for anything that *is* familiar. Elders can insist on "going home," even though they're in the house they've occupied for thirty years; what they really mean is they want to return to where things made sense. Some wandering may just reflect poor short-term memory, leading an elder who thought he or she could just walk to the store and back to get lost. Wandering is among the most common reasons for moving someone to an assisted-living dementia care facility.

Loss of Inhibitions

Damage to the frontal lobes of the brain can remove social controls, reasoning and courtesies that have been a lifetime in the making. When affected, elders may misinterpret social cues. They can become convinced that caregivers and staff members want to be romantic or misperceive the intentions of someone trying to bathe them. They may touch people inappropriately, try to kiss a stranger or fondle a caregiver.

They may say things that they would never have said in the past. They may make tactless comments, create scenes at family gatherings, or start yelling out in the supermarket. They may burst into tears or become upset for reasons that may be difficult to understand.

Sensitivity is the key in these situations. We must help them navigate. We can keep them engaged, perhaps taking them to the opera or a grandchild's school performance. Music is healing to the soul and calming. When that doesn't work, there can be walks in the park. When going out of the home or facility is too much, we can have music and picnics at home. The schedule for an elder with dementia may seem sparse to the daughter who would prefer to do more, but multiple activities in a day may be tiring later in the disease. A chance to rest for an hour or so will lead to a more enjoyable dinnertime.

Compulsion

Some dementia produces repetitive behaviors. Some patients call out a name or just "Help, help!"—only to have no requests when the caregiver responds. Just as the caregiver leaves the room, the calling resumes. Others pace. Still others endlessly sort their junk mail. They may ask the same questions over and over and over. These behaviors are best addressed with engagement. Find things for the elders to do; purpose is important. Ask them to help sort socks, sweep, set the table, fold linens, garden in raised beds, or sort screws or spare change. Of course, other ideas include playing music that the person—not the caregiver—prefers, gentle massage, playing balloon volleyball, going for a walk, or even just holding hands. Sometimes the key is to treat pain. Long-acting Tylenol, 650 mg, three times a day, may take the edge off and not sedate. (Always review with your doctor before using any medical treatments.)

Depression, Apathy, Withdrawal

Some people with dementia may descend into apathy, refusing to see anyone. They may sit indoors with the blinds drawn and watch TV all day or all night. They may start refusing to participate in activities they had once enjoyed. Growing old is challenging for anyone, and it's very common for depression to affect dementia patients at all stages of the disease. Left untreated, clinical depression makes dementia worse. Again, engagement in enjoyable activities is key. If older individuals refuse to accept the presence of a caregiver at home, perhaps it is time to go to assisted living, where they can see others and enjoy the music or art programs. Again the key is engaging activities; it's not fancy décor, but the people and engagement that count.

Sundowning

While research has not pinpointed the cause, people with dementia may become more confused and agitated in the late afternoon and early evening, when the sun goes down. It is a cyclical delirium: Patients may be quite sociable every morning but start crying for their mother every evening or become terrified for no apparent reason. Patients may become unusually demanding, upset, fearful, or suspicious. Sometimes an afternoon rest or a distraction can help this problem. But sometimes the distress can be so severe that medication, sometimes antipsychotics, may be the answer. To be clear: this isn't anxiety, so anti-anxiety medications shouldn't be used.

Irritability

People with dementia face challenges that would be familiar to a toddler: they have trouble understanding the world and even more trouble getting the world to understand them. Elders with dementia often cannot express their needs and communicate that they have wet underwear, the pain of arthritis, a chill from a draft, or hunger.

Not surprisingly, this can make dementia patients irritable, even prone to tantrums. Of course, they're not children and still need to be addressed with the respect of an adult, but their ability to reason and their impulse control has waned. Damage to the frontal lobes leads to the loss of social graces. These elders react differently to problems than they might have done in earlier years.

"Rule Out" Practicalities

Doctors have a method for narrowing the search for solutions to problems. It's called "rule out," which means to eliminate or exclude something from consideration. A blood test, for instance, can rule out whether signs of depression are related to thyroid disease or another medical problem.

In the treatment of dementia, it's important to investigate whether behavioral problems stem from practical issues. Anger, paranoia, and inappropriate action can have a medical basis, but they can also be traced to a wet Depends, to hunger, to fatigue, or to pain. The elder with arthritis pain may express it as anger. He or she may be annoyed about a neighbor's yelling, a bladder that will not empty, or serious constipation that hurts. If a man repeatedly tries to crawl out the window of his nursing home room, is he having hallucinations or does he not know how to get to the bathroom?

In science, a problem-solving principle is that the simplest explanation is usually the correct one. All the issues covered above should be considered and addressed before proceeding with more involved intervention.

Boredom Causes Trouble

Most people have heard the expression "Idle hands are the devil's workshop" applied to children. I always emphasize to families and caregivers that the lack of something to do can actually make an older individual's behavioral challenges worse. People with dementia need meaningful activities to fill their days.

What this means is different for everyone. Elders with vascular dementia tend to be high-functioning at first, in some areas, but often with very poor short-term memory. (It's common for them to look down on others in a dementia facility.) They may like puzzles, playing cards, or outings to shows. Those with more advanced disease may spend hours on simple puzzles or manipulating simple gears or enjoying music, or they may only be able to engage in an activity for a few minutes before they move on. Gardening, baking with assistance, flower arranging, or going on an outing are great for most elders in many phases of dementia.

The trick is to find the right activity to allow an elder to enjoy what capacities he or she still retains. Don't assume that just because someone has dementia he or she can't do anything. I had one man with early-stage disease who still wanted to take his boat out on the lake. His family didn't want him to do it, even though his symptoms remained mild. Going with someone who could do most of the work would have been a good work-around. In this case, the fears of his family limited this man more than his disease progression. Let your loved one enjoy as much as he or she can, for as long as he or she can. Having assistance will often allow elders to participate in activities they traditionally enjoyed.

The key point is that it's not okay to park someone in front of a TV. If someone sits at home all day with a caregiver who says nothing or gets left in a nursing home common room for hours, that patient may get into trouble, acting out from frustration or boredom. Understandably, this often leads to restlessness, calling out, and sleeping during the day, followed by nurse requests for a sleeping pill at night.

Just the act of sitting without moving for several hours to watch TV may cause agitation from back pain. The leg muscles often become weak and contracted after remaining in the sitting position for hours at a time, increasing the risk of falls. Sitting for prolonged periods also increases the risk of pressure ulcers and blood clots.

The "no-parking" rule continues to be important as the dementia progresses and the elder's connection to reality becomes more fragile. For instance, a person with more advanced dementia who watches a news report about flooding may become convinced that he or she is in danger and act out.

More commonly, the experience of sitting in a room with others and watching TV may overstimulate an older individual. The noise and the commotion can become overwhelming and lead to agitation.

Listening to music, painting, playing cards or dominos, or cutting out shapes from magazines are better alternatives to watching television. Ensure that the elder has frequent food and fluid. Elders have fewer sensations of thirst and hunger and may forget to eat. If nothing else works, I find ice cream a reliable alternative (sugar-free ice cream, if necessary, but watch for loose stool from Xylitol and other artificial sweeteners) that decreases irritability.

While some individuals with apathy and dementia can't be engaged, these cases are rare. It's more likely that the family and caregivers just aren't doing what interests the person now.

Be patient, encouraging, and friendly. What did the elder enjoy in earlier years? If someone took pleasure in woodworking but can no longer handle tools, there is sculpting clay (with supervision; occasionally nonfood items can be ingested by those who don't remember they aren't edible) or "gears-and-wheels" sets for kids that can be put together and taken apart. One woman I treated had loved golf. After she was assisted in playing golf on a Wii video game console, she became much less aggressive.

Boxed In Too Early

Gabe was relatively young, only sixty-nine, and suffered from alcoholic dementia. After his wife's death, he began drinking even more heavily. His behavior became erratic and angry. Twice, he ended up in a hospital with alcohol-related illnesses. Finally, his family placed him in a dementia facility, where the other residents were fifteen to twenty years older.

Gabe balked. He refused to participate in the life of the facility, shunning group activities. Although impaired, Gabe—an avid motorcycle rider—still saw himself as active and independent.

"I only want to get on my bike and go down the coast," he said.

Gabe grew increasingly unhappy, angry, and aggressive. His sons were at a loss for what to do. Allowing him back on the road was out of the question. Balancing the risks against quality of life, the sons asked their father if he'd like an off-road dirt bike. Gabe said he would. His doctor told him he would need to train for it and go walking daily. He got out more, and found he enjoyed other activities.

In the end, Gabe never rode the dirt bike. He lacked the physical strength needed to handle the bike. But the act of taking his preferences seriously turned the corner for this man. He began to go golfing, and his agitation decreased as he became busy with outings.

When Behavior Demands Action

If you've taken into consideration preferences, practicalities, and personal engagement but your loved one is still having problems, what do you do? Behavioral issues may make caring for elders with dementia very difficult. Bedridden patients who absolutely refuse to bathe risk skin problems, and those who refuse to be repositioned every few hours may develop bedsores.

Elders who hit their caregivers or who become so distressed and paranoid that they refuse basic care may need medical treatment.

The standard medical approach to these

problems hasn't changed in many years. The first step is to rule out disease: Is there untreated pain from a bladder infection, pneumonia, or constipation? A rapid change in behavior might be caused by delirium, which would be marked by acute onset, waxing and waning symptoms, inattention, confusion, and change in level of awareness (too agitated or too sedated). Delirium is different from dementia. It is not a disease but a set of symptoms, a syndrome marked by confusion and inattention that is a medical emergency and is more common in people with dementia. The evaluation should be completed immediately, since mortality from delirium can be up to 65 percent.

There are no approved medications for the behavioral symptoms of dementia. The anticholinesterase inhibitors donepezil (Aricept), memantine (Namenda), and rivastigmine (Exelon) may help with delusions and behavior in a few people. However, these drugs will not reverse delirium. Most times, they will not stop an aggressive male patient from slamming his caregiver against the wall or keep an elder woman from repeatedly giving her caregivers the slip. They may decrease irritability and some aggression in 10 percent to 30 percent of those treated.

In unresponsive cases, after behavioral interventions and needs are addressed, it makes sense to discuss the risks and benefits of medication in treating behavioral issues. In my experience, there is a role for powerful medications such as antipsychotics or mood stabilizers such as Depakote. Telling families that "nothing can be done" is not only untrue, it's also inhumane.

CHAPTER EIGHT

Treating Challenging Behavior with Medication

TREATING THE BEHAVIORAL SYMPTOMS of dementia remains controversial. There is a sense in the medical community that dementia's behavioral issues are insoluble. In study after study of medications, the conclusion is that nothing works.

Paradoxically, this has resulted in the common prescription of anti-anxiety drugs like lorazepam (Ativan), alprazolam (Xanax) and clonazepam (Klonopin) for people with dementia. While tranquilizers like these may yield short-term results—improved behavior for a few weeks—they're highly addictive. If used for more than a few days in elders with dementia, the withdrawal syndrome often leads to delirium or worse behavior in elders. These drugs can remove inhibitions, cause paranoia, and increase confusion and falls. The person may be better for a few hours after a dose, but if these meds—particularly Xanax, which is twice as powerful as Ativan and shorter acting (the "crack" of anti-anxiety drugs)—are used more than a couple times a month, they often cause more problems than they solve. These drugs start to produce more agitation, poor sleep, or confusion. That leads to an increased dose of Xanax, which increases the withdrawal symptoms, which leads to another increased dose. It becomes a vicious cycle.

A common view in dementia care is that behavior-altering medications should never be used in the treatment of dementia. In this view, all aggressive or anxious behaviors stem from unmet needs that aren't understood by caregivers. Elders get agitated because something's wrong. Their caregivers aren't doing the right thing. They're in pain. Their family isn't being attentive.

In my practice, I have found that it's often not that simple. Linking all agitation to environmental causes is akin to the now-debunked notion that autism or schizophrenia are caused by a lack of parental warmth. Sometimes behavioral or practical measures won't solve the problem. What if a family is loving and attentive? What if a family is attuned to practical issues and medical needs? What if the elder is still lashing out and uncontrollable? These families didn't cause their elder's agitation.

Some doctors feel there isn't yet enough evidence to establish drugs as part of the standard of care for behavior problems in dementia. There's little conclusive research in this area. Just as most drugs aren't tested in children under six years of age, few pharmaceutical studies focus on complicated medical patients over sixty-five, with or without dementia. In the doctors' view, using drugs in this way is like using cough syrup to treat a case of pneumonia; it doesn't treat the underlying cause of the disease.

A better analogy, in my experience, would be that certain powerful psychoactive medications are like chemotherapy. They're difficult to use correctly, and there is higher risk of harm. However, like chemotherapy, these medicines may relieve serious symptoms. Psychoactive medications might mitigate paranoia or delusions that can lead elders to assault others, injure themselves, or live with serious distress that makes their days miserable. In these cases, the medication can restore quality of life. As with chemotherapy, the elders should be followed closely to assure the use of the minimum dose needed for the least amount of time.

However, with careful follow-up, most elders can have symptoms relieved—less pain, distress, or aggression—but remain alert, not sedated. When I prescribe psychoactive medications to treat the behavioral symptoms of dementia, I am trying to make my patients' lives better. I am trying to allow them to enjoy as much of life as they can for as long as they can.

Not treating these behavioral problems robs the patients and their families of the healing that can allow quality relationships. It keeps the elders in a constant state of fear and panic. When dementia patients are antagonistic—claiming they're being held prisoner, that their spouse is unfaithful, that all their food is poisoned, that their children are trying to control them—everyone suffers, the elders most of all.

Treating behavioral symptoms can improve patients' lives, but that doesn't mean there aren't trade-offs. Make no mistake: these are strong medications that can carry difficult and serious side effects. They're not approved by the U.S. Food and Drug Administration (FDA) for use in dementia. These psych medications, particularly when used incorrectly, may cause documented harm: sedation, aspiration, dehydration, weight loss, blood clots, and pressure ulcers from the sedation. It's extremely common that behavior medications, particularly the Xanax and Ativan type, lead to overtreatment and sedation, The key is to reassess the situation every few weeks and start tapering the medications when the elder is alert and engaged. It's never okay to wait for them to go facedown in their lunch to make a medication change.

I believe antipsychotic drugs are worth the risk, if carefully monitored for psychotic symptoms of paranoia and delusions. This isn't a matter of giving patients a pill so that doctors and caregivers have a better day; it's prescribing medications to make the patient's life better. When relieved of anxiety, delusion, compulsion, paranoia, and anger, dementia patients can live more fully in the moment. When behavior symptoms are treated, loved ones and caregivers do not need to be on edge, accused of being jailers, or always wondering when the next outburst or crisis will hit. Aggression, anger, and paranoia decrease. Patients can enjoy their friends and family.

It is also worth noting that many facilities will refuse admission or evict elders with difficult behaviors. I have heard it said that some elders with aggression "will just need to be put in mental institutions." Most often, behaviors can be addressed with behavioral and medical interventions to allow a person with dementia to stay at a more homelike facility, closer to family. Usually, effective treatment involves treating pain adequately and stopping the use of drugs that make the behavior worse, though it may take months to slowly remove the offending medications.

The treatment of pain has become more controversial as well. The Centers for Disease Control and Prevention (CDC) has advised that narcotics should not be used in patients with chronic pain. I trained at an inner-city public hospital and cared for my share of drug- or alcohol-addicted people. I have been threatened over medications. But that was a different population from elders with severe, bone-on-bone arthritis or spinal stenosis. As with other areas of medication use, we use the most simple solution first—a tablet of long-acting acetaminophen (Tylenol) two to three times a day, every day. (As with all medications, check with your loved one's doctor since liver damage can sometimes—but rarely—be a contraindication to its use.) Yes, Tylenol should be given every day for someone with known pain and arthritis. I like to say, "Dementia does not cure arthritis."

Someone who had pain before dementia likely still has it but may not be able to locate the source of the pain and may just become more irritable. Caregivers and nurses are more likely to reach for the Ativan or Xanax for the irritability than the Tylenol for the pain causing the agitation, but I suggest you try the Tylenol first.

I'm always up front with families about the

risks of using strong psychoactive medications. When families have tried every physical, social, and medical treatment available and still their elder remains extremely hostile, paranoid, or delusional, they often decide to take the chance. Here are examples from my practice.

- Maggie's husband, Joe, started having symptoms of early onset dementia in his early sixties. At six foot, four inches and 240 pounds, Joe was extremely strong. When Maggie finally had to place him in a dementia unit, he was extremely agitated. He would throw a bundle of his clothes over the facility fence, then try to scale the wall. He grew so upset and so violent that Maggie had to hire a one-on-one caregiver just to watch him.

  After several weeks adjusting to a new medication regimen that included antipsychotics, Joe stabilized. He required 3,000 mg of valproic acid (Depakote) and 800 mg of quetiapine fumerate (Seroquel). He was not sedated, but he was not as aggressive, and he could finally be engaged in activities for a short time. After several stable months, the doses were decreased to the point that he was somewhat aggressive. That showed what dose he required.

Then we increased the dose slightly. This increase lead to calm, engaged days. His wife and son could visit without him charging the door when they left.

"I hate to think what would have happened if we had not been able to get his behavior under control," Maggie told me. "He would have had to have been locked up, restrained, and heavily sedated. It would have been a very sad ending."

- Barry's mother, in her eighties, became so out of control that even several grown men could not subdue her. When she came to see me, she was on a cocktail of medications, but they didn't seem to help. With some trial and error, we were able to find a combination of drugs that calmed her down.

"There is no way my mother could have been treated without these meds," Barry told me. "My mother wasn't doing well on the normal drugs that a regular physician who doesn't deal with elders prescribed."

- Kyle's mother started to have memory problems in her early sixties. She fought her family and her medical team at every turn. Her dementia pushed her into a state of constant fear. She saw her own reflection in the mirror and thought someone was stalking her. She took a big metal spoon and broke every reflective surface in her room. She stabbed a caregiver with a pen. She broke the furniture. She overturned her bed. She frightened the other residents and the caregivers. She had been treated with increasing doses of Ativan and quetiapine fumerate (Seroquel). The Ativan was very slowly tapered, and the Seroquel was replaced with a small dose of olanzapine (Zyprexa) and valproic acid (Depakote).

Once we changed her medications, she wanted to see her children and grandchildren. Kyle told me, "She thought we were the enemy, but she didn't realize we were trying to help her. With the right medication, she became calm, not sedated, and wasn't afraid anymore."

- Andre, in his eighties, was horrified when his wife of many decades, Emily, became so violent that she had to be taken from her dementia unit in handcuffs, escorted by police officers, because she was a danger to herself and to others.

  "We had tried all the standard medications, the Alzheimer's medications like Aricept and Namenda, but they didn't seem to be helping much," Andre told me. "Your way of handling her case has given her back to me. I lost her. You helped her to overcome some things, not completely of course, but enough so that I could visit her." Emily did not tolerate any antipsychotic medications. However, a small dose of methadone for her severe hip pain and some gabapentin (Neurontin), which also helps with muscle, skeletal, and nerve pain, and a little valproic acid (Depakote) helped to allow her to stay in the facility near her husband without being sedated or in pain.

Finding the Right Combination

Treating these symptoms requires a measure of trial and error, which is typical in other fields of medicine as well. I emphasize to the families of my patients that there is no way to be absolutely sure of finding the right combination of activities, behavioral intervention, pain management, and medications that will lead to calm engagement without side effects. But we can't reach that desired balance if we don't try.

Some of these methods involve the prescription of drugs for uses other than those approved by the FDA. This is quite common in medicine. For instance, doctors may use gabapentin

(Neruontin) for the treatment of joint pain or anxiety, while it is only officially approved for treating
shingles pain. Older, less-expensive medications
such as Neurontin are not cost-effective for any
company to test and market. That said, not all
off-label uses of medications are beneficial to
patients. Ideally, doctors would only use FDA-
approved medications. But in cases where no
medications are approved and the studies do not
point to a reliable treatment, educated estima-
tions and close observation have served patients
well.

Informed consent is crucial. Each family
should know of the risks, benefits, and alternatives of any medication and should be aware if
a medication is not FDA approved. The person
starting any medication should be monitored
closely, and if there is any new symptom, the
medication may need to be stopped to determine
if it is the source of that symptom before more
medications are added to treat the new symptom.

This is a common scenario, particularly with
Parkinson's medications such as Sinemet (car-
bidopa/levodopa), which increases dopamine to
allow better movement. However, it also is more
likely to lead to psychosis, paranoia, delusions,
and aggression. I have seen Parkinson's treated
with risperidone (Risperdal), an antipsychotic
that decreases dopamine, but makes Parkinson's

stiffness worse. And so it goes, with increasing doses and other medications, trying to find the right balance. The right answer is to stop the medications that make Parkinson's disease worse. In my opinion, risperidone should never be used with Parkinson's. Any Parkinson's medications that have adverse side effects should be tapered to the point that the elder cannot function as well, and then increased a little more to allow function. Medications should be reassessed periodically.

Doctors prefer to stick to "evidence-based" medicine, treatments that have been proven effective by studies. The problem is that there are few definitive studies of the behavioral symptoms of dementia patients. As practitioners, we can easily see if behavior improves. But it remains difficult to quantify that improvement in an academically rigorous way. In addition, as previously noted, the use of lorazepam (Ativan) or donepezil (Aricept) may affect behavior, and some studies use them while testing the new medication. Other studies withdraw all psychoactive medications. Unfortunately, as we discussed earlier, rapid withdrawal of the benzodiazepines (Xanax, Ativan, Klonopin) can lead to withdrawal agitation or delirium, which is confused for agitation of dementia.

Definitive direction from studies is still years away. Yet, so many of our loved ones need help today. And the number of those living with dementia increases each year. Ensuring comfort, addressing needs, and providing meaningful engagement are always the go-to options. However, when they fail, I have seen these medicines make a huge difference in the lives of my patients, allowing them more comfort and bringing peace to their families. I have also seen these medications abused, used to sedate, without a lot of thought about the underlying cause of the behavior. To be clear, it is never acceptable to leave an elder sedated. Medications must be reduced and adjusted.

Medical practitioners, families, and caregivers should closely monitor patients who use these medications. Even if a person with dementia remains calm, the team needs to remain alert to possible problems: constipation, decreased interest in food and fluids, poor balance. The goal should be to use the gentlest medications that work and to reduce the dose when possible. I find that after a few months with stable behavior, many people can reduce the amount of behavior medications that they take.

Adjust, and Then Adjust Again

A middle-aged couple struggled with the husband's mother, Pam. In her eighties, the woman's body was strong, but her mind had become clouded. After a reaction to a seizure medication, she became uncontrollable.

One night, she became so combative that six firefighters, three policemen, three paramedics, the facility staff, and her family all converged on her room to calm her. They failed. (Having so many people in a room can make matters worse, but this occurred before I met her. I would advocate for a calm, gentle presence of one or two people if possible.) Eventually, Pam became so disruptive that she was forced to leave the facility.

The family was prosperous and tried to provide the best care available. Pam seemed physically comfortable; she had access to good food and to activities that might engage her. She had patient, trained caregivers. Yet nothing worked. The family didn't know what more they could do.

When I saw Pam, I knew it was going to be a trial-and-error process. She could no longer communicate, so she couldn't tell me what she was feeling. Was she agitated because she was angry and paranoid? Or might she be agitated because something was annoying her?

As possible medical and physical irritants were ruled out, I started adjusting her medications. She had a history of arthritis, so I first tried the long-acting acetamin-ophen (Tylenol), one tablet three times a day. Then a small dose (100 mg or less) of Neurontin, once at night, then twice a day. She was still aggressive to her caregivers, refusing needed personal care, despite the caregivers being patient and trying different approaches. Pam did not like help in the bathroom, but she could not clean herself and was at risk of skin breakdown. In sim-ilar cases, I usually begin with a low dose of an antipsychotic like quetiapine fumer-ate (Seroquel), then wait to see if the patient responds. If the response is not good, I try another. It took a few months, but eventu-ally I hit on a complicated regimen that sta-bilized Pam.

Now, she functions well enough to live in a board-and-care home a few blocks from her son. She can go on short trips with her son and daughter-in-law. She can go out to lunch. She can go to the movies. She is liv-ing in the moment, and living well. It just took time, some patience, and the right combination of medicines.

All drugs have pluses and minuses. While it's important for families to know medication basics, be sure to discuss these options in detail with your doctor. Remember that as a disease progresses, it usually makes sense to taper down most medications. This is especially true if someone is hospitalized; often when elders are sick, they become more sedated from the medications they had been stable on previously. Again, with any sedation, the sedating medications need to be reduced and possibly stopped.

The Case Against Tranquilizers

Would you give Grandma a shot of whiskey to keep her from calling out? Tranquilizers work the same way alcohol works. In fact, they're used to help wean patients from alcohol use. Doctors soften the withdrawal symptoms with drugs like lorazepam (Ativan), alprazolam (Xanax), or clonazepam (Klonopin).

Tranquilizers, like alcohol, can't be stopped suddenly, cold turkey. If a person with dementia takes a tranquilizer for more than a few days, suddenly discontinuing the medication may cause agitation, even delirium. In people with dementia, medical professionals often attribute this distress to the dementia itself or to a medical issue like an undiagnosed bladder infection. Overtreatment of presumed bladder infections is a whole other problem in care of elders. In my experience, in most cases the tranquilizers are to blame.

My first rule for coping with the behavioral symptoms of dementia is this: Don't prescribe any medication that's likely to make the patient *less* inhibited. Many anti-anxiety drugs do just that, damping self-control. Tranquilizers act very much like a couple shots of booze.

In my opinion, we are far too liberal with tranquilizers for elders.

The tranquilizer Ativan is prescribed to millions and is completely accepted by the medical orthodoxy. Nearly one-third of the elders taking Ativan have long-term prescriptions, mostly given by primary-care doctors.

Nearly 5 percent of Americans take sedating tranquilizers in the Ativan or Xanax family, according to a study in the journal *JAMA Psychiatry*. That's about 16 million Americans on tranquilizers.

Elders and women are three times more likely to get tranquilizer prescriptions, especially if they suffer from insomnia or anxiety.

Yet tranquilizers are far from risk-free. Ativan use increases the risk of falls, and thus fractures. It can cause addiction, increased confusion, and aggression. All these risks are greater for older people.

All too often, when someone with dementia suffers with insomnia, they are treated with tranquilizers such as zolpidem tartrate (Ambien), triazolam (Halcion), temazepam (Restoril), lorazepam (Ativan), alprazolam (Xanax), or clonazepam (Klonopin). These drugs have been shown to result in decreased brain function. Tranquilizers may lead to oversedation, increasing the danger of falls. If they are used for a few months and the person develops a tolerance, agitation may then increase. Often, the dose is increased and the cycle begins again. Or the withdrawal delirium looks like worsening dementia. These drugs may even make patients psychotic and less socially inhibited, like someone bruising for a barroom brawl.

Tranquilizers have their place for emergencies. If the elder becomes violent, a tranquilizer may be the only solution. Short-term use in a hospital may sometimes make sense so that a needed test or procedure can be done.

But why is this person in the hospital? It's very common for elders with dementia to be afraid of hospitalization. I sat in the ER with Stan, an eighty-four-year-old man I had helped bring in after being called to his home and realizing he was delirious. As I sat there, the tech said the cursory, "We need to draw blood and do an EKG," and he started to take Stan's arm, tie the tourniquet on, and poke him. Stan pulled away, and the tech held harder. Then the EKG monitor leads were put on without a word. The tech left, and Stan took them off.

People with dementia don't understand the strange routines of a hospital, the hustle-bustle, the scary machines, and unfamiliar sounds. Are we improving quality of life for dementia patients by hospitalizing them? Or are we distressing them and exposing them to drug-resistant bacteria that they wouldn't encounter at home? If patients pull out IV lines and fight with the hospital staff members, they're likely to be tied down and sedated. Is that the goal that we set for care?

Stan died three weeks later in the hospital. He had a bladder infection, which was treated, but the doctor would not release him unless he could sit up calmly on the edge of the bed. He fought the care and was restrained at his wrists and with liberal doses of haloperidol (Haldol). He was stuck in bed the whole time and then aspirated. I had lobbied to get him home with two sets of caregivers, but I did not have the last word.

Many of my patients do not tolerate hospital care well. I provide almost all care at their homes. Much-needed care can be supported at home, from podiatrists, nurses, even dentists. X-rays, blood samples, even infusions can be done at home. And when the end is near, hospice care can also take place at home, where elders feel comfortable and safe.

When All Else Fails

The director of the dementia unit had reached the end of her rope. She had trained all of her staff members in the correct techniques for handling aggressive patients. Her caregivers knew how to go slow, how to be friendly. Over decades in the field, this director had earned a reputation for compassionately handling even the toughest patients. Yet nothing worked with one eighty-year-old man. No matter what the staff members did, this patient continued to slam aides and nurses against the walls. The director contacted the man's doctor, asking for help.

The doctor, who cited his training in caring for dementia patients, sent the unit director a note. In it, he said that medications were not indicated in the treatment of dementia. The staff members on her unit, he wrote, just needed to love the resident.

The next day, the man slammed another resident, an eighty-four-year-old woman, against the wall. He had to be sent to the hospital because he was a danger to others.

Sometimes love isn't enough.

Better Alternatives

Use the following sections for reference as you design a strategy with your doctor.

The challenge is this: Everyone's body chemistry is slightly different. Everyone has a different situation and a different history. Elders are very different from one another in their response to medications. Two people may look the same. They may have the same level of dementia and have similar symptoms. Yet they may react very differently to the same drug. If you've seen one person with dementia, then you've seen one person with dementia.

The key is to know where to start and then be available to hear feedback and adjust strategy. Only then can behavioral symptoms be eased so that life "in the moment" can be pleasant.

Trial And Error to Find the Sweet Spot

Mary is eighty-four years old and recently got kicked out of her nursing facility. She yells, refuses to be moved, and is somewhat sedated with Ativan and a little Haldol. Her daughters report that she has been a difficult woman for a long time.

Upon further discussion, they report she has had spinal stenosis for more than eight years. As her dementia worsened over the previous two years, she has begun to have problems walking.

I stop the Haldol and taper down the Ativan. Mary remains irritable and refuses care. I try gabapentin (Neurontin) and pregabalin (Lyrica), but they do not work to relieve Mary's pain or mood. I try mirtazapine (Remeron), but it does not calm agitation,

After discussing the risks with her family (2 percent increased stroke risk, 1 percent increased sudden death risk), I prescribe one-quarter tablet of methadone at night.

Mary has less pain, is allowing care, and after increasing to one-quarter tablet twice a day, she has the other psych meds tapered down and enjoys her days.

Antipsychotics

All antipsychotics increase the risk of stroke and sudden death, as I've noted before. Obviously, then, they shouldn't be used for behavior that is merely annoying, such as restlessness, simple insomnia, or repetitive questions or actions. Again, behavioral interventions are always first; engagement, comfort, addressing needs. Several antidepressants—citalopram (Celexa), mirtazapine (Remeron) or sertraline (Zoloft)—make much better first choices in cases of anxiety or aggression that haven't responded to other interventions.

Antipsychotic medications are the meds to use if a patient is severely paranoid or delusional. If the patient has extreme anxiety brought on by delusions, antipsychotics can be helpful as well. Each medication has a different effect. Risperidone (Risperdal) is less sedating but rarely causes more stiffness or restlessness (akathisia, which is Greek for "inability to sit"), and quetiapine (Seroquel) is more sedating and rarely causes more confusion, but it may be less effective at treating paranoia.

If one fails, another may work. As previously discussed, they all have a 2 percent increased stroke risk, a 1 percent increased sudden death risk, and all can affect walking. Occasionally, the drugs may interfere with swallowing and may lead to further decline. Try to use the minimum amount necessary for the shortest time possible.

Here are the antipsychotic medications most frequently used.

- **Risperidone** (Risperdal) can help reduce paranoia and delusions. However, it may sedate an elder at higher doses or cause restlessness or akathisia. Because it may cause stiffening or trouble walking, particularly in those with Parkinson's disease (which causes those same problems), those patients should always be given something else, often **quetiapine (Seroquel) or clozapine (Clozaril)**. In some cases, risperidone has been associated with what are called "extrapyramidal symptoms," strange movements or twitches of the mouth or body, another reason it should be avoided in patients with Parkinson's disease.

- **Haloperidol (Haldol)**, an older medication, may alleviate delusions, hallucinations, and paranoia, but it causes extrapyramidal symptoms in 30 percent of those treated, also restlessness, walking problems, and general stiffness. This medication should also be avoided in patients with Parkinson's disease; it is dangerous in that the person can become immobile. This drug stays in body fat for some time, so effects often linger even after the drug is discontinued.

- **Aripiprazole (Abilify)** may decrease hallucinations and agitation without sedating patients. But because of the way the drug works, some patients may actually experience more agitation while taking it. The only way to know is to try it. However, we do not use this antipsychotic often as other alternatives are better tolerated.

- **Ziprasidone (Geodon)** may also be used to treat hallucinations and delusions. There are some reports that it may not be as effective as the other antipsychotics above, but sometimes it may work when others are not tolerated.

- **Quetiapine (Seroquel)** may help moderate paranoia, delusions, and hallucinations, but is less potent than Risperdal (risperidone). It is less likely to cause side effects like involuntary movements or stiffness. Because of this, Seroquel remains a better option for those suffering from Parkinson's or Lewy body dementia. Side effects can include sedation and lower blood pressure or, at times, more agitation because of the drug's anticholinergic effects.

- **Olanzapine (Zyprexa)** may also treat paranoia and delusions. However, it can also increase levels of blood glucose (dangerous for diabetics) or lipids (dangerous for heart patients). However, it may be helpful when Risperdal and Seroquel haven't worked.

- **Clozapine (Clozaril)** is a drug typically used to treat schizophrenia and bipolar disorder. It can be difficult to use: for each weekly supply, a blood test is required to confirm that white blood cell counts remain normal. However, this drug can help some patients, especially those with Parkinson's dementia, who haven't responded to other medications.

Sometimes You Need to Change the Situation and the Meds

Larry, an eighty-year-old man, went into the hospital with mild dementia. As he was being treated for a stroke, physicians had to insert a catheter to drain his urine. He didn't understand why it was there, and he kept trying to pull it out. The hospital staff had tied him down to keep him from doing this. He had become completely incoherent, delirious, not eating or drinking well, and spent all of his time tied to the bed.

When he left the hospital, his dementia had become many times worse, and he was incredibly upset about the catheter. Several times, Larry would pull out his catheter. This sometimes resulted in severe bleeding and a return trip to the hospital. At times the bleeding became so bad Larry needed a blood transfusion. It became a vicious cycle. The family begged the doctors to remove the catheter, but the medical team told them it wasn't possible because the patient was too ill to undergo general anesthesia. They prescribed sedatives and anti-psychotic medications to help him cope.

When I first saw Larry, he was completely delirious. He didn't know where he was. He didn't know what was happening. His family was desperate.

I helped the family to schedule tests that could tell us if a simple procedure (a laser TURP) might make his catheter unnecessary. We found a surgeon willing to do this procedure with spinal anesthetic, rather than general anesthesia. I tapered down Larry's tranquilizers and prescribed a small dose of Risperdal. He was back in street clothes just a few days after his surgery, happier, more alert.

In this case, a combination of addressing the catheter problem, moving him out of the hospital where they would not take definitive action, and changing his medicines helped this man to get out of crisis.

"He's my sweet Dad again," his daughter told me

Sometimes Only Antipsychotics Work

Margo, an eighty-six-year-old woman, started to decline quickly after her husband died. She moved in with her daughter and son-in-law, who had run a senior center for decades. Even with the couple's experience in the field, the family struggled: One night, Margo snuck out of the house at 1:30 A.M. with a bag full of potatoes, costume jewelry, and a remote control. Another time, with two people watching her, she still managed to slip out of the house. She would become agitated, then aggressive, then delirious. She refused to eat. She stayed up all night and then slept all day.

The time came when Margo had to go to the hospital for treatment of a bladder infection. The staff there heavily sedated her to keep her from becoming too disruptive. She was released to an excellent dementia care facility, but even there, she struggled with constant agitation. She tried to escape, fell, and banged her nose. Her family felt confused and upset.

I used a small dose of antipsychotic medication and tapered down the tranquilizers. Within seventy-two hours, there was a turnaround. Her daughter told me she was back to where she had been six or seven years before.

Once Margo stabilized, we tapered down the antipsychotic drugs. She now takes very few meds and has become the social darling on her hall at the dementia facility.

Antidepressants

Understandably, those suffering from dementia may show signs of depression. They may be irritable and edgy. They may not be able to explain their bad mood. They may eat and sleep too much or too little. Early symptoms of dementia may first be diagnosed as depression.

It's important to first address the depression by getting the elder engaged. Sometimes the first episode of late-life depression can be treated with a simple change of schedule or situation: a good day program to end the elder's isolation or the removal of stressors such as an alcoholic, abusive grandson who lives with the person. Or if behavioral interventions do not work, perhaps a prescription for the appropriate antidepressant will work. Not all antidepressants are alike; some may make the elder more agitated, resulting in insomnia and confusion. It's crucial to find a physician who is aware of the challenges of treating older individuals because medications may have more adverse effects on older people than on younger patients.

Just a few decades ago, treatment for depression was limited. Luckily, we live in an age where there are many drug options for easing depression Most of these medicines work by affecting the supply of or the absorption of key brain chemicals.

The largest group of the newer antidepressants are selective serotonin reuptake inhibitors (SSRIs). These drugs work on serotonin, a chemical that helps carry messages in the brain. The drugs block nerve cells from absorbing serotonin, thus increasing the supply of this important nerve transmitter. SSRIs may cause stomach upset or diarrhea and may decrease the sodium levels necessary for health. They may affect walking. For people with dementia, older medications like sertraline (Zoloft) or mirtazapine (Remeron) often result in better outcomes than newer, more complicated drugs. Other drugs affect the supply of norepinephrine, a brain chemical that helps control attention, and dopamine, a chemical key to muscle control and the ability to feel pleasure.

Here are some of the most common antidepressants.

- **Fluoxetine (Prozac)** is the best known and the oldest of the newer SSRIs. It works well in younger adults, but it's not such a good choice for elders. It is very long acting and is likely to dampen appetite, exacerbate insomnia, and lead to irritability and anxiety.

- **Paroxetine (Paxil)**, another SSRI, works for depression, anxiety, and obsessive-compulsive disorder. However, it can be very sedating. It also interferes with choline (is an anticholinergic), resulting in confusion, constipation, dry mouth, and urination difficulties for men. It's likely to exacerbate behavioral problems and can be difficult to discontinue. It's usually best to taper it off very gradually, and it may be better to give it at night and lower the dose if withdrawal symptoms prove difficult. I do not prescribe this medication for older individuals.

- **Citalopram (Celexa)** selectively inhibits the absorption of serotonin. Since its patent has expired, it is very affordable. Some studies have concluded that citalopram decreases agitation, but it doesn't work for all patients. The side effects (as with all SSRIs) include a possible decrease in sodium, stomach upset, and diarrhea. This drug often causes sedation, so it makes sense to take it at night. Still, it's a better choice than a tranquilizer like lorazepam (Ativan), unless a patient needs to be sedated or restrained right away to treat dangerous behavior or is unresponsive to other interventions. Beware that SSRIs, particularly citalopram, can increase heart rate and that in combination with antipsychotics, antibiotics such as ciprofloxacin (Cipro), and certain other medications, SSRIs can lead to serious heart arrythmias.

- **Escitalopram (Lexapro)** is functionally similar to citalopram. This medication can also be sedating, so it's better given in the evening. Its side effects are similar to those of citalopram. Some believe this is a more effective medication, but results vary.

- **Sertraline (Zoloft)** also selectively blocks serotonin reuptake. It's less sedating than related formulations, and it can help those struggling with sleepiness. It is also good for those who may be eating too much, which is sometimes a symptom of dementia. On the flip side, it may "rev up" some patients, leading to insomnia, irritability, stomach upset, diarrhea, and decreased appetite.

- **Mirtazapine (Remeron)** works mainly on the receptors for serotonin and norepinephrine, another neurotransmitter. It's particularly good for patients suffering from anxiety, poor appetite, and insomnia. In the older patient (those who are over eighty years old or frail), it may cause more walking and balance problems than SSRIs. However, if the patient is no longer walking, this isn't an issue. Occasionally, this medicine may cause liver inflammation. Recent studies show it is not as affective for severe agitation.

- **Venlafaxine (Effexor)** improves mood by blocking the reuptake of both serotonin and norepinephrine. It can cause heart stimulation and blood pressure elevation, and its side effects—insomnia or irritability—may worsen in elders. However, it may help patients for whom an SSRI isn't enough, and it can be more energizing than other drugs. One neurologist calls it "rocket fuel." It should only be prescribed in consultation with a trained geriatrician or geriatric psychiatrist. There is also a risk of withdrawal syndrome if the drug is discontinued, so it should be tapered slowly.

- **Duloxetine (Cymbalta)** also blocks the reuptake of both serotonin and norepinephrine. Reports of patient experiences are mixed. This seems to be the flavor of the year, touted as a treatment for pain. However, my patients with pain have not had significant relief, and I spend much of my time tapering it down or discontinuing it because it can cause more agitation and poor sleep. It may also cause headache, dizziness, insomnia, nausea, and constipation, among other side effects. It can be complicated to use because of side effects and withdrawal issues.

- **Bupropion (Wellbutrin)** may help those who are eating too much or feeling more lethargic or apathetic. This drug may energize patients, reduce appetite, and cause insomnia. It shouldn't be used in those at higher risk for seizures.

In some cases, elders taking antidepressants to treat agitation may instead become more agitated and restless, and they may suffer more insomnia and emotional unpredictability. This may be a side effect of the medication or the symptoms of bipolar disorder. One of my patients, Ralph, had appeared depressed with his hip replacement, so he had been given Celexa. One day Ralph disappeared and returned with a new car! Our psychiatrist helped stabilize his previously undiagnosed bipolar mood disorder with valproic acid (Depakote), and the car was returned. A psychiatrist should be consulted in these complicated situations.

Radical Treatment, Radical Improvement

Bonnie was an eighty-six-year-old woman who was withdrawn, apathetic, and had been diagnosed with advanced dementia. In the past, she had suffered an episode of severe depression and had responded well to electroconvulsive therapy (ECT), once known as shock treatment, to trigger changes in brain chemistry. We tried this treatment again. The woman did so well after ECT that she was able to move from a dementia unit to a structured, assisted-living facility. Yes, that is an unusual story, but ECT and other treatments should be thought of in select cases.

Mood-Stabilizing Medications

Some elders may become quick to anger or have serious mood swings that don't respond well enough to multiple trials of various antidepressants. In some cases, there's simply not time to wait three months or more for symptoms to change when a patient enters another stage of dementia. Another group of drugs called mood stabilizers may yield results in these situations.

Prescribing these drugs for dementia patients remains controversial. These medications calm nerve function. When first introduced, they were used to treat seizures. Later, physicians realized that they could be useful in treating schizophrenia and bipolar disorder, once called manic depression. They help with mood swings, insomnia, accelerated or frenzied speech, and grandiosity ("I just talked that over with the President" or "I'm going to buy an airplane tomorrow").

The FDA has not approved these meds for use in dementia patients, yet they are prescribed off-label. A discussion of the risks and the benefits is essential in order to give informed consent. If they are used, it is best to start at low doses.

- **Valproic acid (Depakote)** can be very tricky to use with elders who are frail. However, for a patient who is climbing walls, trying to escape, and physically lashing out at family and staff, someone who is quick to anger, this drug can ratchet back the aggression where other medications have failed.

There are risks in using this drug. The biggest risk is that it can affect balance for frail elders who are walking. Rarely, it can cause liver inflammation or lower blood cell counts. It should be administered at the lowest dose possible for the shortest time. I've found that it's best to look at the patient's behavior to determine quantity (usually starting with 125 mg once in the evening, or less). This is a key point: to use only the minimum dose, rather than follow a conventional therapeutic level that is standard in treating bipolar disorder, which often results in oversedation (and the resultant increased risk of falls, aspiration, blood clots, pressure ulcers, dehydration, and sleep cycle disruption).

It may irritate the stomach. It can never be crushed, but comes in sprinkles and liquid form. Both physicians and caregivers need to monitor the patient carefully. When the elder is doing better, that's the time to start tapering off.

- **Gabapentin** (**Neurontin**) was originally developed to treat seizures and is FDA approved for the treatment of shingles pain. However, it has been used off-label to treat the nerve degeneration known as peripheral neuropathy, joint pain, and anxiety. When the nerves that carry messages to and from the brain and spinal cord don't fire correctly, the result can feel like burning pain and numbness

While peripheral neuropathy can happen to anyone, I have treated many patients in long-term care who have abused narcotics or tranquilizers. I found that gabapentin avoided addiction issues and helped calm a wide variety of patients: one man with post-traumatic stress disorder who had to stay in the hospital to receive IV antibiotics for six weeks, another who suffered from terrible sciatica, another who had spinal pain.

The most possible side effects of gabapentin include; sedation, rare confusion, constipation, dry mouth. Most elders tolerate this drug pretty well, and it has fewer serious effects than long-term Xanax or lorazepam (Ativan).

- A similar, but more expensive medication, **pregabalin (Lyrica)**, is FDA approved for treatment of fibromyalgia. It may be more effective for nerve pain and is less sedating than gabapentin, but again, some people may become more confused.

Likewise, I have found that gabapentin can effectively calm some people with dementia, where behavioral interventions are not enough and when another doctor might reach for the Ativan. It may decrease anger and anxiety for some; for others, it may do little but make them sleepy.

- **Carbamazepine (Tegretol)** is used by some, but it has not been shown to relieve symptoms in most patients and leads to serious sedation. This drug also has many side effects, including liver inflammation and decreased cell counts.

Daughter Held Hostage

In her middle age, Penny leaves her home in New York to help care for her mother, Kathy, in Detroit. Kathy can't take care of herself, but she won't accept any caregiver except for her daughter. Kathy's needs swallow up the daughter's life. Kathy grows increasingly paranoid and aggressive, but she will not allow anyone else to help her at home. This goes on for years.

Several times, when the mother is hospitalized, Penny asks to have her placed in a care facility. Penny has reached the end of her rope. She can't go on taking care of her mother without help, but her mother vetoes outside caregivers. Yet each time Penny asks, the social workers at the hospital just send the mother home.

The first step to softening the mother's paranoia and anger employed ice cream— with a small dose of valproic acid (Depakote) and olanzapine (Zyprexa) mixed into it because the mother wouldn't take pills whole. Most facilities are reluctant to take on disruptive elders, but with medication, Kathy's behavior calmed down, and it became possible to place her in a facility.

Five years on, the mother is smiling more, takes only a small dose of Zyprexa (which when stopped leads her to refuse all care and medications), and is engaging in activities with other residents. Penny was able to reclaim her life, and she is relieved knowing that her mother is well cared for and enjoying her days.

CHAPTER NINE

Living with Dementia: Coping Day-to-Day

ADJUSTING TO A DEMENTIA DIAGNOSIS can be frightening, frustrating, and difficult for both the family and the older individual. It's important to remember that there's lots of help available and that having clear goals, adjusting routines, and using a few simple strategies can make the journey much smoother. This chapter will outline some steps that will make life with dementia easier. Some of these tips, I have developed over years of experience, but many come from facility managers, medical specialists, and other professionals.

First, Heal Thyself

For family members, dealing with their own feelings may be one of the most difficult tasks. They must cope with their own pain, anger, frustration, and fear. Families often feel overwhelmed with questions: Why did this have to happen?

Why do I have to deal with this huge hassle? How can I overcome my own grief now that my parent, spouse, or sibling seems to be slipping away? If my relative suffers from dementia, will it happen to me?

These feelings are completely natural. I see them again and again, in family after family. Until you recognize these feelings and begin to process them, you won't be able to effectively help your loved one. Seek out a support group or other family members. Look for books to help you work through these feelings. See the "Resources and Further Information" section at the back of this book for suggestions.

Stephanie Howard has worked with dementia patients and their families for almost twenty years. She has worked for several residential care companies, managing memory communities around San Francisco and running family support groups. Howard is passionate about patient-centered care.

Here's her perspective on the emotional toll that dementia takes on families.

"Where do you start? First, you get a box of Kleenex. There's a lot of anger and pain just after a dementia diagnosis. I always think it's better to get all that out in the open, to just cry together. After you get past that, you are more able to gain ground.

"You have to ask yourself: Are we talking about how the dementia is affecting the family? Or are we talking about how the dementia is affecting the patient?

"Families are worrying about lots of things: Many times, it's a monetary problem. How long is the money going to last? How long is their elder going to live? Often, these aren't answerable questions.

"Meanwhile, the person with dementia is struggling with different questions, depending on how far the dementia has advanced. In the early days, they may worry about the loss of the future they thought they had. Later on, they may simply express anxiety when things change. The point is, the elder's problems are often very different from the family's."

The Elder's Point of View

One of the things that can be so frustrating about interacting with a person who has dementia is that it seems so uncertain, so uneven. It's like walking on shifting sands. Elders may still remember how to make a meal but struggle to sign a check. They may forget directions from five minutes ago, but remember a childhood Christmas. Or elders may seem physically hale and hearty, still exercising and moving well, but become unable to manage some of the higher thinking skills necessary for organizing finances or a household. Loved ones may become angry, anxious, paranoid, suddenly promiscuous, or unusually shy. They can be annoying. They may follow family members around like a lost puppy. They may ask the same questions over and over again. They may be overconfident and stubborn one minute, hysterically afraid the next.

If it's difficult to manage this terrain as a family member, imagine what it's like for the person with dementia. In its early stages, dementia can be terrifying. Try to remember back to a time when you lost something important, like your wallet. Remember that dread and terror, that pit in your stomach as you imagined someone merrily charging up the balances on your credit cards? Now imagine that you have that disorienting, catastrophic experience one hundred times an hour. That approximates what life is like for many with dementia as their disease first becomes noticeable.

For people living through the onset of dementia, things that once were easy have suddenly become difficult. They often feel lost. As the world becomes ever more confusing, they worry about losing control, about being "found out." Because they don't want people to see their diminished capacities, they often stop seeing friends. They make excuses. They avoid activities they once enjoyed. Some know that their abilities are slipping and feel useless, ashamed. Some, especially those with vascular dementia, have brain damage that blocks their self-awareness. They think that they're fine and that the worried family members are crazy and trying to take control of them. They may become withdrawn and depressed. In other cases, the apathy and loss of empathy aren't symptoms of depression but of the dementia itself.

They may become suspicious. They forget where they put their watch and conclude that someone stole it. They start hiding their jewelry, forget the hiding place, and become sure that someone is stealing from them. Their children are stealing their money. (This may be true, but often is not.) They're sure their spouse is unfaithful, or suddenly they may not even recognize their partner. ("Who is that old guy?" a wife might ask, remembering only the young man she married decades ago.) Why are family members keeping them from doing what they want to do?

This is the point at which patients often can't manage their finances, and things begin to veer out of control. Often, the family notices and tries to get the patient to give up control or to at least accept some help. Alas, this usually confirms the patient's worst suspicions.

A Person with Dementia Is Still a Person

As crazy-making as the onset of dementia can be for everyone, it's key to remember that people with dementia have feelings. They have needs and wants, just like anybody else. They enjoy good food. They want to make choices about what they wear, eat, and do. Yet those with dementia may not be able to voice their desires. For this reason, it's extremely important to provide doctors and caregivers a full history of the loved one so that they can understand the preferences and routines the elder had before being diagnosed.

It's also important to remember that people living with dementia aren't children. They're full-grown people who need to be accorded the respect due adults. While their abilities may be failing, they're still grown-ups.

Too often, people make the mistake of treating someone with dementia like a child. This may be because people with dementia have much in common with children who haven't yet developed abstract reasoning and judgment. The elder's abilities are changing and uncertain. A lot of things seem strange, unexplained. The world seems alternately exciting and threatening. For this reason, it may be helpful to employ some of the same techniques that work when parenting children.

- Remember to smile and to be reassuring.

- Do not yell at or belittle the elder.

- Give one-step instructions.

- Give the elder time to process each request, each step in a process.

- Give simple choices. Not "What do you want to wear?", but "Would you like the red shirt or the blue shirt?"

"The elders are our educators," Howard says. "They tell us what they want and how they want to be cared for. We have to have open ears so that we can understand them.

"Task-oriented care never works with dementia," Howard says. "It always has to go back to the person. Do you find yourself touching the person with dementia? Maybe that person doesn't want to be touched at that point. You need to ask questions, get their opinion, let them make choices if they can. It's important to remember not to do what you think you should do for them, but do what the elder would want to have done."

Howard works to engage residents at whatever level works for them now. Here are some of the tricks of the trade that she's developed.

Steps to Structure

As scary and disconcerting as dementia is to elders, a simple, well-defined structure for daily life can help ease their fears. Knowing what's going to happen each day builds a feeling of security. In the beginning, providing reminders of the day and date can help lend structure. Later, when they no longer care, let it go.

Be open with elders about what's happening to them. As anybody knows, the monster in the closet is always far worse than the one you can see. Let them know that there are things they can do to slow the progress of their condition. Answer their questions.

If they refuse to acknowledge that there is any problem, don't insist on making them recognize what's happening. Work around it. Build the structure they need. Help them keep as much of a sense of independence as is safely possible.

Allow more time for everything. You may be on a schedule, but the person with dementia isn't. If you're stressed about time, your loved one will pick up on it and may become angry, even belligerent. Take it down a notch. Let things get done in their own time.

Find a way to keep the elder socially active. This may be a club, a day program, a class, a regular card game, or a weekly get-together with family and close friends. Some do better with a one-on-one companion to take them out for a few hours a day. Others like groups. Studies show that social connection and interaction help preserve mental function.

Provide opportunities for physical activity: walks, gardening, golf, balloon volleyball. While motor abilities vary widely among elders, studies have confirmed what your grandmother said: a healthy body nurtures a healthy mind. Elders, even those with dementia, who exercise regularly experience a slower cognitive decline. They're also less likely to fall, break a bone, and become bed-bound. Tai chi has also been shown beneficial for all elders.

Break tasks into small steps. Do not ask the elders to hurry and get dressed, shave, and come to breakfast. That is a recipe for disaster; they'll get lost in the first task. One step at a time: Put on your underwear. Put on your pants. Put on your socks. Put on your shirt, and so on. Be patient. Do things in the same order each day. This minimizes anxiety and makes success more likely.

Avoid saying *no*. It just creates conflict, and fighting isn't really fair or productive when your opponent has dementia. This doesn't mean giving in to every whim. Rather, it means thinking about what motivates your loved one. With finesse and creativity, you may be able to inspire him or her to do the things that need to be done.

Mirror the attitude you want the elder to have. As some senses fade, others become more acute. Those with dementia are often highly aware of and sensitive to the moods of others. If you're cranky, your loved one's mood will suffer as well.

Make sure to offer choices. If your mother constantly asks, "What are we going to do?" ask her, "What do *you* want to do?" Give her choices. Opening the closet and asking what she wants to wear confronts her with an overwhelming number of choices. Rather, ask if she feels like wearing the red skirt or the blue skirt. Either-or questions work best.

Let the small things go. If your father or your husband shows up at the holiday dinner table wearing a striped shirt and plaid pants, does it really matter?

Don't hesitate to walk away if things get strained. Come back to the idea of bathing, or whatever's causing conflict, in half an hour. Failing that, ask another caregiver to step in. Or if that's not possible, "change your face." Sometimes just changing your clothes or putting on a hat or a pair of glasses will alter the dynamic enough to allow the person with dementia to make a fresh start and successfully handle the task at hand.

Try to laugh. Dementia inevitably creates funny situations. Let your loved one know that you forget things, too. Make it safe to forget: Lose your keys on purpose and then point out your mistake. Let elders know that they're accepted, and laugh *with* them when things get goofy.

Personal Care Strategies

For someone with dementia, the daily routines of physical maintenance eventually become a challenge. Elders with Parkinson's disease and Lewy body dementia develop coordination difficulties earlier than some others because those diseases affect muscle control. But elders with alcoholic or vascular dementia and Alzheimer's eventually struggle as well. Establishing routines can help to keep the patient as functional as possible, for as long as possible.

Timing is important. Someone who's always stayed up until 3 A.M. and slept until 11 A.M. is not going to want to be up and dressed at 7 A.M. A man who has always showered in the morning isn't likely to be willing to switch to evening baths. A schedule often can be adjusted some, but do it slowly.

What If a Patient Won't Wash?

Ask a person with dementia, "Would you like to have a bath?" and it isn't at all uncommon to be told, "Thanks, but I just had a bath." You may get this response even if the patient hasn't washed in a month.

The elder may also see the suggestion as an affront to his or her independence. The refusal is just another way of saying, "I can take care of myself, thank you very much!" Or it may be that the patient just doesn't remember or doesn't perceive the dirt and the need to bathe. As brain function falters, so does perception. Sometimes elders resist washing because bathing is just sensory overload: Think of all the feelings, the sounds and smells involved—the person has to be naked, likely cold, may not like the feel of the water landing on the skin, some other person there, "watching."

If your loved one resists bathing, change the subject for a while and then try again. Try to make bath time as calm and appealing as possible. Make sure the room is warm, the elder is covered with towels that can be removed and replaced as parts of the body are washed. Giving the elder a hand-held showerhead and letting them do most of the washing can also help. Yes, that means water spraying around and wet towels, but so be it. Consider a sponge bath as a half measure until you can get the elder into the shower.

Romancing the Hairdresser

One of my patients had always been an elegant dresser. For most of her adult life, she'd had her hair styled at Elizabeth Arden. She'd worn designer clothes and fancy Italian shoes. As her dementia progressed and she became bedridden, she suddenly refused to bathe or to have her hair washed. It seemed shocking for someone who'd always cared so much about her appearance.

After weeks of pleading and wheedling, her caregivers got her to agree to a sponge bath several times a week. But the patient held firm on washing her hair. The most she would permit the caregivers to do was brush her hair with dry shampoo powder, a half step at best.

This continued for two years, until one of the caregivers had a flash of insight into the woman's stubborn resistance. The patient had always had her hair done at a high-end salon. She didn't want just anyone to wash and style her hair. She wanted a professional. But she was too weak and frail to go out. The caregiver called a nearby salon and asked if a stylist would be willing to make a house call.

When the "expert" arrived, suddenly the

woman's objections to hair-washing disappeared. She cooperated as the stylist
washed, cut, and dried her hair. Weekly
appointments with the stylist followed.

Strategies for Bathing

To help your loved one keep to a routine of bathing, it may help to prepare a calendar to hang
on the wall and mark off certain routines, like
bathing and social engagements. Make it fun:
say something like, "Every Tuesday and Friday
is shower day, and then we'll have a treat." Link
the shower with going to the salon to have a cut
and blow-dry or to a round of golf or a visit to a
favorite restaurant.

Remember that bathing brings into play issues
of modesty and dignity that are much more central to older generations than they are to many
of us who are younger. Use towels to cover parts
of the body that are not being washed at the
moment or avert your gaze to make the patient
as comfortable as possible. Have an unbreakable
basin with a washcloth that the patient can use
to bathe himself or herself. Having a sturdy bath
seat and not leaving the elder alone unsupported
is key to preventing injuries.

Try to make all the externals pleasant: Make
sure the room is warm. Have all the towels,
soaps, and lotions set out and ready. Remove

bath mats or floor towels, which can increase the risk of falls. Quiet music, lemon-scented room freshener, or a bowl of potpourri may have a calming effect.

Magazine advertisements for a walk-in tub may look appealing: just open a door on the side of the tub and get in as if it were a taxi. However, this requires people with dementia to sit naked for a long time until the water fills up around them. For many people, replacing a bathtub isn't practical.

Using a European-style handheld shower-head and a bath seat is another option to make it easier for the patient to bathe independently. I myself prefer a bath, as do many older individuals. However, if an elder has mobility limitations or lack of judgment, having a bath in a tub is very difficult, sometimes dangerous. If in doubt, ask an occupational therapist to do a home evaluation to see what approach is safest.

Remember that older skin is dry skin. Bathing with just warm water for most of the body is just fine. For other areas, use a gentle soap such as Dove or Basis, and apply lotion afterward.

Strategies for Dressing

Your aunt may never have left the house without being dressed to the nines; your father may seem naked without a business suit. But this isn't the stage of life for formal, complicated clothing. Zippers, belts, hooks, bras, long rows of buttons—all these can make dressing an ordeal. Also, elders often have very dry, very fragile skin. Tweeds, wools, stiff linens, and other fabrics can cause irritation.

Look for fashionable alternatives in soft fabrics. The key words should be *soft*, *warm*, and *comfortable*. Garments should be easy to put on and take off. For women, camisoles may be a good alternative to bras. Stretch pants are a godsend.

Let the patients choose between a few options in what they wear. Have everything ready before you start. Make sure the room is warm. Remember that it may be stressful for elders to get naked. Hand the elders a towel for cover or hand them their underwear and be as unobtrusive as possible and still be safe.

Be very aware of the elders' dignity. Don't do something for them without giving them the opportunity to do it independently. Don't step in unless they really can't do it themselves. It may take longer, but it's important to keep them engaged and as independent as possible; it slows the decline.

Strategies for Eating

Dining should be a pleasure, but as dementia progresses, the mechanics of eating become difficult. Keep breakfast flexible, according to personal preference, but make sure lunch and dinner happen at predictable times.

Try to avoid late-night meals, as this can exacerbate gastrointestinal reflux and heartburn. Late-night snacks may also increase the risk of aspirating food into an airway. Fluids after dinner may increase the need to urinate at night and make insomnia worse.

Caffeine should be avoided, as it can cause irritability, insomnia, and frequent urination at night. If elders wake in the middle of the night, give reassurance, perhaps a sip of water, and return them to bed; avoid giving them a snack or putting on the TV. Screens at night lead to more insomnia and should be avoided; try peaceful music instead.

Pay attention to the little things. If at all possible, have the person with dementia help decide on a menu for the week. Take care with how the food is presented on the plate. Remember that smell can boost the appetite. Simmer cinnamon sticks or vanilla beans in a pot to create a pleasant ambiance.

Avoid alcohol. It dampens the senses and further handicaps people whose cognitive abilities are impaired. It also leads to more insomnia and agitation and hastens mental decline. If your mom has always had a glass of cabernet with dinner, pour her some nonalcoholic wine without comment. We have also had success putting that nonalcoholic wine in an empty bottle of a previous favorite, for the brand appeal. If the elder refuses to go along with this, water down wine and serve it in a small glass. For cocktails, I would advise to slowly water them as well, first by 25 percent, then 50 percent, then 75 percent for a small shot, and when unnoticed, stop the alcohol. Then enjoy the evening ritual this person has kept for the last forty years.

As dementia progresses, it becomes more difficult to coordinate the use of knife and fork. There are many things you can do to allow elders to feed themselves as long as possible. One good tip is to try to use the weighted silverware designed to help Parkinson's disease patients suffering from a pronounced tremor.

Remember that many forms of dementia affect vision and depth perception. Technically, a person's vision may be fine, and yet the image communicated to the brain may be incorrect. In this case, the patient may have trouble knowing exactly where the plate is in space. Make sure the color of the plate contrasts with the table. A white plate may get lost on a white linen tablecloth. Appropriate contrast will help get the fork where it needs to go.

With more advanced dementia, starting to

eat may become difficult. This is damage in the parietal lobe that helps guide sequencing: sock before shoes, time to eat when you are given a plate of food, and so on. You can help your loved one by placing your hand over the hand that is holding the fork of food, helping the person keep eating mostly on his or her own.

Eventually, utensils will become too much of a bother, too much to handle. Then it's time to switch to finger foods: chicken nuggets, sliced vegetables and fruit, cubed ham, triangles of toast.

Drinking is as important as eating. Liquid keeps the blood chemistry balanced, flushes out toxins, keeps the bowels regular, keeps blood pressure and energy up, and does many other vital jobs. Caregivers must provide frequent opportunities to drink. Elders may not perceive thirst or hunger and may only take a sip when a glass is offered. So it needs to be offered often. A healthy elder should drink enough to urinate at least every six hours. As stated earlier, it is best to avoid caffeine because it is a diuretic and will frequently lead to insomnia and urination at night.

Elders eventually are going to have more trouble swallowing. Make sure the elders tuck their chin in and swallow twice after each sip if they are starting to show signs of a problem. If you have any concerns, have a speech therapist evaluate the patient and provide instructions for safety. You may be advised to chop food or add nectar to thicken fluids. You may be advised to start using a sippy cup. Toward the end stage of dementia, the swallowing reflex fades altogether. At that point, your loved one will stop swallowing. That is a sign that the elder is very near the end of the disease. Of course, all medications that would oversedate should be eliminated before this stage is diagnosed.

Strategies for Toileting

Toilet routines often conflict with very strong feelings about dignity and modesty. To maximize the likelihood of success, ask a physical therapist or an occupational therapist to do a home evaluation to determine the best place to install a grab bar or the proper height for a commode with arms that will fit over the toilet. Medicare often covers these evaluations.

Give plenty of opportunity for bathroom breaks. It's normal for most people to need to use the facilities about thirty minutes after a meal. Make sure this timing becomes part of the daily routine. When accidents happen, don't draw too much attention to them. Just say, cheerfully and matter-of-factly, "Oh, you've had a spill! I think we need to change those clothes, don't you?" If the person with dementia is still somewhat high functioning, give him or her a choice of what to change into.

When a patient begins to lose bladder or bowel control, a good strategy is to schedule a bathroom visit every two hours. It is hard to have an accident if your bladder has just been emptied. Sanitary pads may be helpful as well. For those who can no longer empty on command, disposable briefs are the best choice.

When "pull-ups" do become a necessity, don't make a big deal about it. Just get rid of all the underwear and say, "We're going to use these now." Calling pull-ups "disposable underwear" makes them less of an issue.

Constipation is an issue that needs to be addressed. It can cause agitation, loss of appetite, and poor sleep. Occasionally, being plugged up may cause a life-threatening bowel perforation. People with dementia often lose track of the last time they had a bowel movement. As dementia slowly erases body awareness, they may not understand that the pain in their lower abdomen may signal that it's been too long since they last had a bowel movement. Bowel habits need to be monitored to make sure patients have a bowel movement about once a day and don't have to strain. It's harder to move one's bowels when lying down than when sitting on the toilet.

It is important that everyone drink enough fluids, eat fruits and vegetables, and keep walking and active. However, with dementia, the range of acceptable foods may narrow dramatically. In the worst case of not wanting to eat, I find that most everyone will accept ice cream (or the sugar-free, lactose-free equivalent) and Boost, Ensure, or Carnation Instant Breakfast drink mixed in beverages, or smoothies.

Generally, I avoid prescribing fiber treatments such as Metamucil or Citrucel. With these solutions, the stool turns to concrete if the person doesn't drink enough, and forgetting to drink is typical of those with dementia. MiraLAX is a better choice—it draws water into the gut—but one must drink water with it or you just get a pasty mess. Senna and magnesium tabs are also good choices if constipation is an issue. Although magnesium is billed as critical to other health functions, almost no one needs supplementation. However, this is one area that magnesium really can be helpful.

Sorbitol or xylitol, common agents in sugar-free products, draw water into the gut. Most people will enjoy sugar-free candies, puddings, or ice cream, and the sorbitol or xylitol in these treats will help keep them regular.

Check the Bowels

In my experience, it's often prudent to begin the search for a patient's complaints by ruling out constipation.

Paul, an eighty-seven-year-old man, complains that he can't urinate. That often happens when the prostate gets compressed. His caregiver takes him to the emergency room. There, the doctors do an abdominal CT scan. They find that the poor man's colon is firmly packed with feces. His bowels are so plugged up that the blockage has pinched off his urine flow. He's more in need of a rectal exam than a CT scan.

I see this happen again and again. The rectal exam is the only way to really tell if someone is very constipated. You can't pat someone's abdomen and really know how the bowels are functioning.

Strategies for Dental Care

With all the other health issues facing elders, dental care commonly gets lost in the shuffle. A catastrophic illness may shoulder its way to the top of the priority list, forcing dental care to the bottom. As it becomes more difficult for the elder to get around, cleaning appointments may fall by the wayside.

As long as the elder is brushing and not complaining of dental pain, families may think there's not a need for a dental visit, especially one that might be difficult for the elder and the family. Meanwhile, as motor skills or health awareness falters, the simple act of brushing teeth may become difficult for the elder, but having someone else do it may seem an invasive ordeal. So elders and families often avoid dental issues.

This is a mistake. Even if someone has had lifelong, consistent dental care, a lapse in maintenance can lead to rapid decay that makes extractions necessary. You may not see cracks around that bridge, crown, or denture, but they're there. These microscopic openings allow bacteria to slip in—bacteria that will establish themselves in those cracks and rot the teeth.

Dr. Peter Y. Kawamura is a San Francisco dentist who's part of a growing group of dental professionals who make house calls to elder patients who can't travel to a dental office. He uses miniaturized equipment to perform almost any procedure found in an office setting. He often works with patients in various stages of dementia. He shared some tips for handling dental care for elders with dementia.

According to Kawamura, the first line of defense is daily brushing. Websites like www. specializedcare.com sell all kinds of tools to make this easier. Buy a three-sided toothbrush (Benefit, Surround, or another brand) that scrubs the front, back, and crown of each tooth in one stroke. The brush may look odd, but it will cut down on brushing time and reduce stress.

As patients become unable to care for their mouths, caregivers should gently take over the task. Buy a dental prop. This wedge-shaped soft device keeps the patient from biting you. Go slowly. Explain what you're going to be doing. Let the elder look at the instruments you will be using and try them out. Don't try to clean the entire mouth in one sitting. Each time, try to clean just a bit of the mouth. Let small successes build on each other.

It may be helpful to hook thumbs with the elder and hold the toothbrush à la chopsticks or a pencil grip. With the hooked thumbs and the caregiver guiding the toothbrush, the person will be alerted by the movement of his or her own arm that something is coming to the mouth, and the elder may be less startled. This technique can also be useful for feeding elders who can no longer feed themselves.

It may also help to make the room feel as much like a dental office as possible: Recline the bed to an angle similar to a dental chair. Put on a face mask. Wear a camping headlamp that's reminiscent of a dentist's headlamp. All these props will likely stir memories of being in a dentist's office and may inspire the appropriate behavior. Or that may not work at all; each person is different. Try several approaches until something works for your loved one.

Don't forget to make appointments with a real dentist at least every six months. This is especially important after a long illness or hospital stay. During these emergencies, patients may go a month or more without brushing their teeth. A professional cleaning is in order as soon as possible. Dr. Kawamura also recommends regular oral debridement by a dental hygienist or dentist and regular periodic application of silver diamine fluoride (SDF) applied to all root surfaces of teeth to minimize/stop tooth decay and promote the longevity of dental restorations.

If getting to the dentist has become an ordeal, look for a dental hygienist or a dentist, like Kawamura, who will make house calls. Some dentists will do so for long-time patients. A few will do more involved procedures at home. Investigate whether your area has any dental hygienists in alternative practice. This specialty includes hygienists who work independently of a dentist's office, and many of them do house calls.

Strategies for Hospital Stays

The hospital can be a scary place for anyone, but it's especially so for someone suffering from dementia. Imagine having an operation when you have no context, no understanding of what's happening to you. Who are all these strange people rushing around? Why are they poking me with needles? What are these tubes in my arm? Why do I feel pain? What are those voices, and what are they saying? What are those beeping sounds? Why is my bed rolling down the hallway? Why does everything seem so fuzzy? Why can't I go home? Why is everyone telling me to stay still? All these questions and the fact that elders perceive pain differently create terrible anxiety for most dementia patients.

I'll never forget accompanying a friend to outpatient surgery. The elder woman in the next treatment bay obviously had fairly advanced dementia. A middle-aged woman, her daughter I guessed, answered all the preoperative questions. The problems began in post-op. The elder woman woke up from anesthesia crying out for her daughter. Unfortunately, that hospital only allowed visitors to stay a few minutes in the crowded post-op ward. The poor woman cried for her daughter for hours. She was hysterical by the time she was released to go home. Often in these situations, patients receive heavy sedation. They're then discharged with a much higher risk of falling, breaking bones, or aspirating food.

Sometimes awful incidents like that can't be helped. But they raise questions about how certain situations fit with the goals of care. What makes life worth living? If the elder can understand that he or she is getting help for a medical problem and doesn't fight the care, then hospital treatment may be fine.

But what if the elder doesn't understand why he or she is in the hospital? What if the treatments seem like attacks—tying down the elder to put in an IV infusion or, worse, putting a catheter into the bladder (which to some may feel like a sexual assault).

I always advise families to consider what adds to improving the quality of each day. If an elder is scared, can't comprehend the treatment, and fights back, how does that improve quality of life? For some, it is better to stay in their "home" with its familiar surroundings and familiar caregivers and to receive as much treatment there as possible. When the elder has declined to the point that he or she qualifies for hospice (a prognosis of six months or fewer), hospice teams can help support the elder at home and attend to comfort.

If your loved one must be hospitalized, families need to make sure that each doctor, nurse, and orderly knows that your relative has dementia. Try to set up a schedule of familiar people so that someone trusted is with the person with dementia at all times, both to answer questions from medical staff members and to minimize the loved one's anxiety. If you have a musician in the family or a good storyteller, sometimes playing tape recordings of familiar voices will take the edge off the anxiety.

Have a list of habits, medications, and concerns ready for the doctors and nurses. What medications is the elder taking? What behavioral concerns does the elder's regular medical team have? What things does the elder find particularly distressing? The more information you can give the hospital staff, the better.

Some families also find it helpful to post a short letter to the staff and to tape it to the head and foot of the patient's bed. The text may read something like this: "Dear Staff: My mother has dementia. Please speak slowly. She'd like to understand but she can't. We love her very much and hope you will give her the best care possible."

CHAPTER TEN

Getting Help:
Options for Families

THROUGHOUT THIS BOOK, you've read again and again that the goal should be to preserve as much function as possible for as long as possible. Families are, and should be, central to this effort. But there are many different professionals who can help families achieve this goal. Just as it takes a village to raise a child, it also takes a village to care for an elder with dementia. In this chapter, you'll find an outline of the types of specialists who can help your family and your loved one.

Occupational Therapists

Occupational therapists deal with the practicalities and the techniques for helping patients preserve and improve their quality of life. They form a bridge between medical concerns and social concerns. Julie Groves is an occupational therapist based in the San Jose area, with decades of experience in consulting with patients and families in their homes. She shared some things all families should know.

Occupational therapists ask questions that are different from those that doctors ask. "Instead of asking, 'How do we fix this illness?'" she says, occupational therapists ask, "'How can the elder get back to having a good life?' 'How does this person adapt?' 'How can this person accommodate the mental and physical changes they're experiencing?'"

Occupational therapists work out personalized systems and adjustments that allow patients to continue eating, bathing, dressing, toileting, socializing, and all the other things that make up a fulfilled adult life. Sometimes this may get done in one or two visits. In other cases, the occupational therapist may check in more regularly: every few weeks or every few months. Medicare usually pays the cost of an occupational therapy consultation for identified events, such as falls risk, hospital stays, ordering a wheelchair. For wheelchairs, always ask for a reclining wheelchair and a gel cushion to decrease the risk of pressure ulcers from sitting in one spot all day.

It's often impossible to teach new things to a confused person, so occupational therapists try to figure out how patients can get what they

need with the skills they retain. The most successful solutions do not remind or correct, but
give help without the elders realizing that they're
being helped. In addition to cutting down on
arguments, this attention to subtlety will also
bolster the elders' self-esteem. It can be difficult to remember all these different techniques
in the moment. Ask the occupational therapist
to write down the protocols. That way, caregivers at home or in a facility can institute changes
to make daily care better.

In dementia care, occupational therapy almost
always centers on working with family members
and other caregivers. How should the furniture
be arranged to allow for maximum freedom of
movement? If bath time is a battle, might it be
because the person with dementia is afraid? If
Dad isn't eating, would he get better nutrition
if snacks were set out on the counter to remind
him to eat?

Dementia often affects parts of the brain
that initiate tasks, areas that help us plan and
carry through. This is called executive function.
Your mom may no longer have the brainpower
that prods her to start a meal or even to ask
for one. In addition, she may have lost the ability to sense hunger. Don't wait for her to say
she wants dinner or ask, "Do you want dinner?"
Just announce, "Here's dinner!"

Dementia may also damage the midbrain, which is thought to coordinate all the sensory input that we receive. Keeping the daily routine the same can make it easier for those with dementia to "go with the flow" and enjoy the day. Conflict over routines may have roots in some sensory problem, rather than in stubbornness.

Occupational therapists also help devise systems to ward off problems that inevitably develop as dementia progresses. Assume that your loved one is going to fall. Assume that your loved one is going to make a bad decision. Assume that your loved one is going to have fear about day-to-day tasks. Anticipate caregiver burnout. It's easier to cope with these difficult issues if you have systems in place at the beginning.

Physical Therapists

While it's important for those with dementia to keep moving, periodic hospital stays or other chronic conditions often strand them in bed. For every day elders spend in bed, they lose 5 percent of their muscle mass (That's 50 percent in ten days!). If the person with dementia is hospitalized, ask for a physical therapy evaluation as soon as your loved one is admitted. More than once I have been called to the cardiac unit for an elder who came in for heart failure or arrhythmia, stayed in for five days, and now cannot walk (yes, that fast). Even after just a couple of days, it may require a physical therapist to help an elder get going again. You can also call a physical therapist when a loved one does not seem as steady on his or her feet as before.

Physical abilities need to be constantly reinforced. You need to use your body, or your body will become less and less fit. Sitting in front of the TV all day is the worst. Much better is engaging in meaningful activities and being active. Tai chi, walking, dancing, and doubles tennis are all great ways to be social and active.

Even if exercise is not possible, it's important to keep working on motor skills. Have the patient roll over in bed. That uses a lot of muscles. Keep your elder as active as possible with fun activities, and the physical therapist can do an assessment and write out protocols to keep the patient safe.

The therapist will work to help the elder walk as independently as possible. The therapist will help determine if a walker is needed to stabilize walking, and if so, which one (so don't buy one on your own). A walker is much more stable than a cane.

People with dementia often have trouble getting motivated to do physical therapy. They may get confused and/or agitated. They often do not remember the therapist from appointment to appointment. Because these situations can be so difficult, some physical therapists avoid treating folks with dementia. I have heard more than a dozen times when referring an elder to a therapist for a history of falls: "Patient has dementia, not appropriate for rehabilitation, patient discharged." Your geriatrician or the local Alliance on Aging should know of therapists who can handle those with failing brain function. The point is not that the person with dementia has to "learn" the skills, but that the physical therapist works with the elder and guides the caregivers on how to safely assist in walking or transfers.

When embarking on a physical therapy program, morning appointments in a quiet environment usually work best. People with dementia are more likely to get frustrated and cranky if they are surrounded by noise or if they are tired in the late afternoon or early evening. Enlist the help of family members and caregivers. A familiar face present for the appointment will give the elder the security to get with the program more quickly and, thus, to get much more out of treatment.

Look for a therapist who knows how to break down complex movements into a series of small, achievable steps. Just as recommended in occupational therapy, have the physical therapist write down step-by-step instructions for helping your elder. People with dementia won't be able to keep long instructions straight. Also, use goals as a tool. For instance, if you want the person to walk a couple steps, say their snack is in the next room. The patient may be more willing to make the effort if there's a payoff.

Care Managers

When caring for a relative with dementia, you may feel like you need to "do it all," but that may not be possible. Caregivers can't always be superheroes. They have jobs, children, and other commitments. That's where geriatric care managers come in. These professionals—often trained as nurses, gerontologists, or social workers—have expertise in dealing with the practical issues of aging.

Care managers can provide a one-time consultation, or they can be helpers who deal with all the details of medical care, social engagement, and home management. They can:

- Assess and make the home environment safer.

- Assess the overall health and well-being of the client.

- Develop a personalized care plan with the input of the client and the family.

- Identify and set up resources that need to be in place, such as home health aides, adult day care, and durable medical equipment.

- Help coordinate and manage various treatments and act as a liaison with doctors and other medical professionals.

- Coordinate discharge planning after a hospitalization.

- Arrange transportation to and from social and religious gatherings.

- Manage household services—cleaning, maintenance, shopping—as needed.

Care managers do not make decisions for families, but they identify alternatives and possible solutions. They do as much or as little as a family desires.

Most family members feel relieved when a care manager becomes part of the mix. The addition of such a helper may make it easier to discuss difficult issues or alternatives. For instance, an elder may be more open to the suggestion of hiring a financial manager if it comes from a "professional" rather than from a family member. If asked, care managers can give advice on elder care issues most families find challenging, such as advance health directive choices or deciding when a dementia community is appropriate.

Studies show that elders who have care managers are less likely to be hospitalized or to visit the emergency room. By making home systems more efficient and by cutting the need for family travel, care managers can also save money in the long run. But care managers may not be right for every family or for every budget.

Care manager fees vary widely, from $100 to $150 an hour in San Francisco to more than $200 an hour in New York City. In some cases, long-term care insurance or the Department of Veterans Affairs will pay the fees. Generally, however, the care manager bill must be paid out of pocket. Some communities have social workers who can help through the local Aging and Adult Services office.

Consider whether your needs are more medical or social. If they're more medical, you might want to choose a care manager with a nursing background. How many years' experience does the person have? What would be that person's initial ideas for meeting your family's needs? Can he or she provide references? The Alzheimer's Association in your area will provide local resources.

Caring for the Caregiver

In most families, I have observed that the role of primary caregiver seems to fall to one person. This seems to have more to do with personality and family dynamics than it does with proximity or convenience. You may live close by or may not work outside the home or may be particularly close to the person with dementia. Or you may work, have children, and live a plane flight away. Whatever the particulars, you need to remember to take care of yourself. Managing the care of a partner or relative with dementia may be one of life's most difficult challenges. It can't be done—not for long, anyway—under conditions of exhaustion, isolation, personal anxiety, and professional chaos. Here are some tips.

- Work at letting go of the guilt. While life with dementia can hold good times, dementia also causes many problems. Accept that some of these problems will never be solved. Don't beat yourself up because you can't make everything perfect. Dementia isn't perfect.

- Join a support group. You can't help your loved one unless you have a safe place to air your own fears, anxieties, and frustrations. Many day centers and nursing homes sponsor them. The Family Caregiver Alliance (www.caregiver.org) offers pioneering resources for those caring for people with disabling health conditions. Disease-specific groups like the Alzheimer's Association (www.alz.org) or the American Parkinson Disease Association (www.apdaparkinson.org) will make referrals. Local chapters of the Alliance on Aging will also make recommendations. These groups provide emotional support, referrals, practical advice, and information about other resources.

- Don't be afraid to ask for help. Caregivers often get so burned out that their own physical and emotional health suffers. When people inquire about how they can help, ask if they can come over for a couple hours so that you can do an errand or just have a little time to yourself. Hire a caregiver to allow several afternoons a week away from caregiving. Studies show that the primary caregiver is much more at risk for illness and death from the stress of caregiving.

- I have seen families where an unspoken decision has been made that only one person will be responsible for all the care of the person with dementia or where there is a blended family with a second spouse and the children from the first marriage. That is a recipe for trouble. A family meeting should be held to clearly spell out the responsibilities and the compensation in some way for the person devoting his or her life to the care of the elder, as well as the finances for care and who will be in charge. I strongly also advise that a yearly review be required for the person in charge of the finances.

- Get educated. There are many, many books out there to help families cope with the issues that surround aging and dementia. See the "Resources and Other Information" appendix at the end of the book for a list of those I think are most helpful.

Sucked Dry

For decades, friends commented on what a devoted couple Monty and Doris made. They met during World War II. He was a handsome GI; she was the sparkling life of the party. After the war, they married, bought a house, had two children, and enjoyed a prosperous middle-class life of socializing, golfing, and travel. But then Doris's mental capacities began to falter.

Doris grew paranoid. A piece of racy junk mail, a Victoria's Secret catalog, was enough to set her off. She accused her husband of cheating. Then she started to get suspicious of her son and daughter. She was convinced that someone was stealing from her. Though she normally had a sunny, loving personality, she began to pick arguments. She didn't want her husband to read the paper. She insisted that he stop subscribing to periodicals. She didn't want him to leave her long enough to do the basic housework. She refused to go to the doctor, and she didn't want her husband to go, either. If he even tried to close his eyes, she'd yell, "Don't you go to sleep on me!"

This went on for months, then years. Though he was miserable, Monty believed that it was his duty to take care of Doris. Not understanding that Doris's demands and paranoia were caused by dementia, he thought Doris's personality change was somehow his fault. He felt guilty that he couldn't meet all of Doris's needs. He put off his children's offers of help and barely managed to keep the household afloat.

Monty persevered, but he was emotionally and physically spent.

Finally, as so often happens with primary caregivers, Monty got sick. His congestive heart failure made an operation and hospital stay necessary. Only then did Monty admit he needed help with his darling Doris.

Sadly, it's all too common for caregivers to drive themselves to collapse before admitting that they can't do it all. Recognize from the outset that caring for a dementia patient is a job that can last a long time. It can sap the strength of the strongest person. Take care of yourself so that you can take care of your loved one.

CHAPTER ELEVEN

Getting Help: Long-Term Care Alternatives

FIGURING OUT HOW TO MANAGE the care of someone with dementia may be one of the biggest challenges a family can face. Deciding on the best care option is a very personal decision. To choose the right solution for your family, you need to consider two major factors: finances and the support system that will help the patient get the most out of life.

If your loved one needs twenty-four-hour care, cost will be a major factor. An assisted-living facility will run $4,000 to $8,000 a month; skilled nursing care (or a nursing home) often runs $10,000 a month. Around-the-clock professional home care costs $10,000 to $20,000 a month. These numbers may be lower in a rural state like Kansas or North Dakota and higher in urban areas like New York City. No matter what your geography, though, care doesn't come cheap. While long-term care insurance will cover some of this cost, most policies will not cover all of it. Medicare and health insurance do not cover these services.

Keeping elders in their home can be rewarding. The surroundings are familiar, and they're likely to be close to those who know them. Some folks are just capable enough that they can care for the basics if family members bring them groceries and take them to appointments, and these people are not ready for caregivers in any form. Others, with a well-trained home care staff, may continue to enjoy outings, shopping at the mall, eating at restaurants, gardening, and socializing with friends. Knowledgeable caregivers are able to gauge the elders' current state: Tired? Hungry? Bored? And with a friendly, reassuring manner, they can address the elders' needs and engage them in activities they enjoy.

So what do you do when your mother is missing meals, not bathing, missing appointments, not changing clothes, and getting more confused at night, but she refuses all offers of help and caregivers? This is a common challenge. Often, from the brain damage, people with dementia cannot see that they are not caring for themselves. They become offended at any suggestion they are not "clean" or are incapable of daily care.

Launching a frontal attack—hiring a caregiver and sending that person in for eight hours or more each day—usually backfires. The elder re-bels, and the "interloper" is sent packing. I have found that the caregiver needs to be introduced slowly, perhaps as a "friend" of the family. It's a good idea to at first have a family member there in order to decrease fear of a new person. Per-haps start at two hours, three times a week for a few weeks, then a few hours daily. Often, the time can be expanded from there. Any medical event with a hospital stay is an opportunity to intro-duce caregivers. You can market the addition of caregivers as a way to get out of the hospital. In that sort of situation, the caregiver is accepted more readily.

People often promise loved ones that they will never be placed in a facility. "Don't worry, Mom. I'll never put you in one of those places." These exchanges are understandable. First off, as the saying goes, there's no place like home. And in the past, the care of those with dementia too often has been institutional and impersonal. At its worst, elder care has been bleak and unsafe. Yet there are increasingly more residential options these days, and programs are steadily improving and evolving to meet modern needs.

Don't discount the possibility that—despite promises that may have been made—remain-ing at home may not be the best option for your loved one. Family members may be too close to the patient to be objective about his or her needs. They also may not have the necessary training to care for difficult behavior related to dementia. Thus, some needs may not be met.

Emotional conflict also gets in the way of providing the best care to the patient. For instance, it is very common for people with dementia to consider the family caregiver a "jailer." The "jailer" tells them what to do and won't let them do everything they want to do. People with dementia may feel lonely and bored, which only leads to more conflict.

In a good dementia care community or vibrant day program, visits, outings, and activities will be part of every day. Quality of life may improve. Family members will be relieved of the physically and emotionally draining aspects of sole responsibility of care. A family can go back to being a family, and professionals can take over the nitty-gritty of the engagement, personal care, and logistics. Families who cannot afford to hire the caregivers at home or cannot care for the elder at home for other reasons should not feel guilty.

It's still very common for people with dementia who live in care communities to say, "I want to go home." That also is a common refrain of elders with dementia who live in their home of forty years. Don't let this send you into a spiral of guilt. When a loved one says things like this, he or she often really means, "I want to go back to when everything made sense." Obviously, that's not possible.

Though it may be extremely difficult, again consider the goals of care: What does your loved one need to be successful? What does "success" mean now? Where can he or she best get those activities and support? Consider also that as dementia progresses, transitions from one living situation to another become increasingly disruptive and difficult. The needs of an elder may change as they age; the sociable assisted living community may be too much when the elder is impulsive and falling often, but not engaging with groups.

Start by getting referrals from the U.S. Administration on Aging's Eldercare Locator (www.eldercare.acl.gov), where you can search by zip code, city, or county. Local offices of the Area Agency on Aging also link to community-based resources.

The following sections offer an overview of the basic alternatives for dementia care.

Day Programs

Staying at home all day can be exhausting and frustrating for both the elder and the caregiver. Day programs offer a middle ground between living at home and being in an assisted-living facility or nursing home. There are many different types of day programs. Some are publicly funded; some are private pay. Some offer a program day that lasts four hours; others go for as long as twelve hours. Some emphasize medical care; others the social and educational. But they all provide a facility where elders come together, socialize, and participate in activities, while some also offer physical, occupational, speech, and other therapies on-site.

Day programs help people with dementia continue to do what they enjoy. If they like building models, they should keep building (perhaps more simple) models. If they like gardening, get them busy with the planting and weeding, though it's key to have raised beds to minimize bending and the risk of falls. They should have social outlets. A diagnosis of dementia doesn't mean people should collapse into a recliner or a wheelchair for the duration. They should keep moving. If tennis isn't realistic any longer, maybe balloon volleyball is. Short-term memory loss doesn't get in the way of dancing. Tai chi is great for community participation and has been shown to decrease falls.

Most families don't seek out a day program until there's a crisis. Perhaps the person with dementia wanders off and is picked up by police. Or perhaps an accident makes it clear that driving is no longer an option. The earlier an elder enrolls in a day program, the better. If the program becomes familiar before dementia becomes advanced, the elder will adjust more easily. The routine of going to a day program adds structure and interest to the passing days. Interaction with others improves mood. Increased activity also contributes to better sleep patterns. For people with milder dementia who still need outside engagement, suggesting that they "volunteer" to help the seniors and work alongside the staff members may be a more acceptable framing of this activity. Speak to the administrator, who is likely experienced and creative in helping loved ones adjust to a new environment.

Most people with dementia initially resist the idea of a day program. "Why?" they ask. "I'm just fine staying at home." It depends. If there is support at home to keep the elder engaged in activities, outings as well as with family, a day program may not be needed. However, too many elders spend their days parked in front of TVs, just watching whatever is on the channel. Sitting for more than two hours at a time increases the risk of pressure ulcers, blood clots, muscle contracture, and weakness of the legs. That increases the risk of falls. The elders may doze during the day and then not sleep at night. Or they may just demand snacks and gain weight, making it even harder to walk. Day programs can give them an activity separate from the family. And as we all know, it is good to be away from the family for at least part of the day.

Suggest that the elder just give a day program a trial period, say two months. I advise a family member to go with their loved one the first week to break the ice. It usually takes less time than that before people begin to look forward to the interaction and the activities.

When you're looking at senior centers and trying to decide which is right for your family, remember to look at it through the eyes of the elder. Your spouse may have been a college professor, and an exercise class that involves throwing beach balls around may seem like something that he or she never would have been interested in, but that activity may be just right for where your spouse is now. Give the program a chance.

Check to see if people are really engaged in activities, rather than just sitting around or wandering the halls. Do the staff members seem cheerful and encouraging? How many staff people are there compared with the number of clients? Laws generally mandate a ratio of eight clients to each staff member, but programs usually keep much lower ratios than that. Many programs run at six to one; Alzheimer's programs at four to one. When calculating these ratios,

be sure that the facility doesn't count adminis-
trators, a common dodge to make it seem that
there's more supervision than there really is.

Day programs vary widely in cost, but you can
expect to pay anything from $50 to $100 a day
depending on location and program. Adult day
health programs receive some public funding
through Medicaid and offer subsidized rates, and
PACE programs (Program of All-Inclusive Care for
the Elderly, a Medicare/Medicaid program) may
be covered by insurance. Laws require that they
have medical staff members on-site, so these
programs generally offer shorter days to contain
costs. Some private facilities may offer a sliding
fee scale based on a family's ability to pay.

Home Care

Some patients may prefer to stay at home or
they may need help at night or they may need
twenty-four-hour care. In these cases, consider a
caregiving agency. Research each company thor-
oughly. Remember, these firms will be sending
people into your home. Check them out the way
you would if you were hiring someone to watch
your newborn child.

What is the agency's reputation? Will they provide references? Are they insured and bonded?
What kind of training do they provide to their
caregivers? What kind of background check do

they do on their caregivers? (At a minimum, they should do a criminal background check and a tuberculosis test.) How are caregivers supervised? Can you meet the caregivers before they're assigned?

Insist on a caregiver who has experience working with people with dementia. Such caregivers will know techniques that other caregivers may not, and they will tend to be more understanding of the patterns and behaviors of these elders. Also insist that the caregivers speak the same language as the patient. If your loved one can't communicate with a Spanish-speaking caregiver, he or she may become isolated and withdrawn, which doesn't add to quality of life.

You may also choose to hire a caregiver privately, which is usually less expensive. Remember, though, that in this case, the caregiver is probably not insured and that you are responsible for all the background checks and other tests. If the caregiver is sick or can't come to work, you must have alternatives. Ask all the same questions you would if you were vetting an agency.

Assisted-Living Facilities

An assisted-living facility is an intermediate step between complete independence and a skilled nursing or dementia community. In independent senior housing, elders must be able to take care of their own medication and medical appointments without guidance or supervision. In assisted-living facilities, often the elders can care for their daily activities, such as eating and walking independently, but the staff members provide the medications, meals, personal assistance, and housekeeping.

Many variations on the theme exist. In the facilities for the most independent, residents have their own apartments. Other facilities have private apartments but communal dining. Still others offer transportation as needed.

Some programs provide more structure and support to allow elders with milder memory decline to remain in the assisted-living area. That may be great for a patient's self-esteem, engagement, and sense of normalcy.

However, if the person with dementia has a tendency to wander or to have significant behavioral issues, other elders will ostracize that person for the odd behavior. In these cases, the elder needs a secured residence for personal safety.

Remember that you aren't picking out a hotel. A facility that has beautiful views, flawless landscaping, and tastefully appointed rooms may not have staff members trained in dementia care. It may not have equally top-notch programs that engage your loved one and help him or her to preserve as much function as possible for as long as possible. It may not have equally excellent food, with attractive fruits, fresh vegetables, and an emphasis on hydration. (Dehydration is very common among people with dementia because they forget to drink. This can cause a whole array of health problems.)

Ask all the same questions about dementia care training, staff-to-patient ratios, insurance, bonding, and background checks that you would for other types of elder care.

Look for a facility that offers stimulation at the highest level possible for every patient. Look for small group activities and individualized attention. Remember that we have a "use-it-or-lose-it" brain. People with dementia need to do things and stay as active as they can. For instance, your father may have been a terrific bridge player but may no longer be able to remember the complex rules of counting cards and bidding. Perhaps he can play a simpler game, like dominos, and be successful at that level. Your aunt may have once been an expert at needlepoint but no longer have the motor skills or the vision to do it. Maybe she can paint on fabric instead.

Board-and-Care Facilities

Some patients and families opt for board-and-care facilities, usually private homes where two to three caregivers take care of five to six patients.

The quality of care varies greatly in such facilities. I have found the best ones are often run by nurses. Be sure to ask lots of questions, do background checks, and get references. A board-and-care facility will not usually have as many activities as a larger one. In some cases, a patient may attend a day program and come home to the board-and-care setting in the evenings.

This type of care can be a good solution if patients have more medical needs than can be addressed in an assisted-living setting, such as they don't drink fluid so they need frequent prompting or they have frequent falls and need to be watched more carefully. It's also appropriate for elders whose dementia has progressed to the point where they can only cope with one person at a time. A smaller, more personalized setting may be less stressful for these folks than a large dementia unit.

Assisted-Living Dementia Communities

If elders begin to wander, if they become aggressive or forget to eat, they may need the more supportive environment of a dementia community. Ideally, these units provide more staff members to look after residents, a physical environment that is easy to navigate, and activities appropriate for those with dementia. Since about 60 percent of residents in nursing homes or assisted-living facilities have some kind of dementia, this kind of facility is the fastest growing segment of the business, according to the Alzheimer's Association.

Unfortunately, there isn't very much oversight of these programs. In more than a third of cases, according to the Alzheimer's Association, families weren't informed before admission that dementia communities are more expensive than regular assisted-living accommodation. Facilities aren't always clear about exactly how the dementia wings are different from other residential areas.

When run well, these units can make life much better for elders. But be sure to ask questions: How much will it cost? What sort of programs does the facility provide for residents? Do staff members receive training that is specific to dementia care? How does the facility handle the problems common to people with dementia? Is the community set up in a way that is safe yet pleasant for dementia patients?

Remember that appearances are not as important as programs and a well-trained staff. Don't choose a place just because it looks like a Hilton and has fancy décor. It's much more crucial to choose a community where elders are alert and engaged in activities and where the staff members are easily found, helpful, and friendly.

Activities and personal interactions are crucial to good care. Spend some time at the facility.

Drop in unannounced. Are residents engaged in interesting activities, or are they dozing in their chairs? Are residents walking around? Beware of any place where everyone is in a wheelchair. That suggests the staff members don't work at keeping their residents walking, which leads to pressure ulcers, blood clots, or the frozen muscles known as contractures. Lately, I am seeing more facilities that are short-staffed. Some elders with dementia wander or even try to run away; they need supervision. Other elders require help with situations such as toileting and left on their own might fall and injure themselves.

Check out the "Dementia Care Practice Recommendations" on the Alzheimer's Association website (www.alz.org/professionals/professional-providers/dementia_care_practice_recommendations). Be wary of any dementia care unit that doesn't meet these basic standards.

Skilled Nursing Facility

Often, families come to me thinking that a nursing home is the only alternative. Nothing could be further from the truth. Few people with dementia need to be in a nursing home. That is the right choice if an elder has been in the hospital and is too weak to go home and if that is the only place to get frequent physical therapy. If the patient needs rehabilitation and can tolerate being in a facility and can follow all the rules, this level of care makes sense. However, if elders are distressed, fighting care, and scared of the intervention, they may do better at their residence with familiar surroundings and caregivers, with a home health physical or occupational therapist and a visiting nurse.

Nursing homes offer much more skilled medical care than other facilities. In these places, there are nurses to help with diabetes care, complex wound care, and other complicated medical issues such as emphysema. The downside is that nursing homes are less homelike and more institutional. They usually offer fewer activities. They do not necessarily provide more attentive care.

Ask all the same vetting questions you would of other facilities: How many patients per staff member? What sorts of enrichment programs are available? How are problems handled? How does the facility communicate with the attending physician and with the family? What are the costs? There is a movement, the Eden Alternative, to help make these facilities less factory-like in part by adding plants, pets, and other homelike touches. If you can, try to find a facility with these amenities. However, again, it comes down to staff concern and commitment, not advertised perks.

Hospice Programs

Hospice programs offer caregiving and medical care in which the goal has shifted. Rather than seeking to prolong life and treat every disease aggressively, the goal of hospice care is to provide comfort for whatever time is left to the patient. Patients are eligible for hospice care when their life expectancy is six months or fewer.

Hospice services can provide incredible comfort and peace at the end of life. Hospice agencies feature an interdisciplinary team of professionals with expertise in end-of-life care. These teams attend to the whole person, not just his or her diseases, offering psychological and spiritual services as well as creature comforts like massage in some programs. Studies have shown that patients who receive hospice care at the end of life have better pain control and are less likely to be hospitalized. Their families report greater satisfaction with end-of-life care. Emotions remain long after many other aspects of someone's personality have slipped away. Hospice programs provide a warm, calming environment that helps both patients and their families.

Hospice care remains underutilized. Too many people end their lives in intensive care units, even though there is no hope of curing what ails them. The average stay in hospice care is only three to four days before death. All of these trends hold true for people with dementia even though Medicare has covered hospice care for dementia since 1982.

Part of the problem is that it's so difficult to know exactly how long a person with dementia is going to live. These elders often decline by degrees, in a process that may go on for years. It's important to remember, though, that dementia is a terminal disease. Even when treated, pneumonia for an elder with moderately advanced dementia has a 25 percent chance of resulting in death. Often, this is because the elder lacks awareness of early symptoms and delays treatment. Those with advanced dementia (loss of ability to move, engage, or eat) are at the end of life.

Families may fear that hospice care is about death. Actually, as a hospice medical director, I found that good hospice staff members focus on life, on making each day as good as it can be, and on helping elders and their families to live in the moment. The approach varies. Beware the hospice that just gives dementia patients a dose of morphine, Ativan, or haloperidol (Haldol) as an easy treatment for agitation.

If it seems like your elder is nearing the end, at least discuss the option of hospice care with your medical team. Of course, each family should make the decision that works for them and that is consistent with the elders' wishes or with what you think your loved one would have wanted. Imagine your loved one's younger self looking down on you now. If you're giving the care you think he or she would want, instead of what you want, you'll have less guilt of "doing the wrong thing."

Nobody wants to talk about the end of life. If at all possible, though, try to have that tough conversation. Does your elder want to do everything to prolong life, or is he or she concerned with the quality of life?

If your loved one can make his or her wishes known, those wishes on the basic issues of life and death should be honored. The woman who can't remember things from day to day wouldn't be in a good position to understand the ramifications of intubation, but she could say if she wanted oral antibiotics for treatable medical issues. The choice of forgoing a treatment that might prevent death is a basic right we shouldn't take from someone who can choose.

One sticky issue is determining if the elder has the capacity to make such medical decisions. Kay was living alone, marginally, but protected her independence. She developed a severe leg infection and delayed care. When taken to the hospital by neighbors, she was told she needed to have an amputation: the leg was too damaged to save. She refused the surgery. An outside local aging counselor was called in and explained to Kay that she would die within weeks if she did not have the surgery. By this time, the hospital had decided she did not have the capacity and could not now choose to have the surgery.

This actually worked out well for her. It would have been miserable to cut off her leg against her wishes. How would she take to having to be in the hospital? Having pain that was not well treated? (Elders with dementia almost never get adequate pain relief...if any at all. They are more likely to get agitation from pain treated with Ativan.) She would have needed to stay in bed, have daily dressing changes that are also likely to be painful. And then there are the complications....

Instead of an unwanted major medical intervention, Kay was placed on hospice, given wound care and morphine for her pain. She died peacefully a few months later.

What is the ethical way to address challenging care questions? First, the hospital should have an ethics board to decide what should be done, after a person's capacity to choose has been evaluated by a neuropsychologist. As covered in chapters 3 and 5, the Mini-Mental State Examination screening test is not adequate to definitively diagnose dementia or mental capacity.

It's most important to remember that elders

should be allowed to make their own choices for as long as they have capacity. If a person changes his or her mind to have life-saving treatment—as long as it has already been advised by the physicians—that person has the right to choose the treatment to live.

We must also remain alert to the overuse of hospice care—of referring elders with dementia to a hospice facility because they've been to the hospital too often. Beware the doctor who thinks that a man with moderate dementia and pneumonia should have the antibiotics stopped and be treated only with morphine at a hospice site, even when the man is getting better and wants to go back to his community for bingo.

CHAPTER TWELVE

Legal Matters: Protecting Your Loved One

MONEY. YOU MAY NOT WANT TO TALK about it, but if you suspect dementia or your elder has been diagnosed with dementia, then you can't avoid it.

First, you need to make sure funds exist to take care of the person. How much is available makes a huge difference in what your plan of action will be. Then you need to make sure that this person is protected from the many, many scams that exist to separate addled elders (or isolated, lonely elders without dementia) from their savings. Then you need to set up systems that make sure the bills are paid on time. None of this is easy, but it's essential.

In earlier, more subtle levels of the disease, people with dementia may remember the day and place where they are but lose judgment or the ability to reason abstractly (think finances). In social situations, these people sound good. But in reality, they should no longer manage their money. These are the people who used to diligently research investments but suddenly put thousands into highly speculative penny stocks because a new broker suggested it. They are people who may allow a new "boyfriend" or "girlfriend" or someone much younger to take over their financial matters.

If someone has the capacity to judge risks and benefits of a proposed intervention, then adults have "the right to be folly." However, if an adult is suffering from dementia and lacks the ability to assess risk, that person needs to be protected from predators.

Every family's situation is different. It's important to consult experts—fiduciaries, elder law attorneys—to help you with the particular details of your case.

Assess Capacity

I can't say this enough: As soon as you think there's a problem, try to have your elder evaluated. Standard tests like the Mini-Mental State Examination (thirty questions such as "What day is it?" and "Draw this pattern") or the Montreal Cognitive Assessment (MOCA) may be a starting point. However, I've often seen elders get passing scores on the MMSE but be completely unable to make a health-care decision or decide whether to stay at home or move. In fact, it is still taught in some medical texts that a score above 24 means there is no dementia and a score below means the person has dementia.

Mental capacity is the ability to make decisions for yourself. The definition of mental capacity is the ability to understand information for a decision, weigh the risks and benefits, and communicate the decision to others. Bear in mind that certain medications (including acetaminophen [Tylenol PM, which also includes Benadryl], lorazepam [Ativan], alprazolam [Xanax], and other sedating drugs) can make people seem more impaired than they actually are. Testing should be done after the medications are removed. (Sleeping pills and antianxiety pills need to be tapered slowly.) For early, less obvious cases, it's much better to get more comprehensive neuropsychological testing instead of an opinion from a family doctor or the local neurologist or psychiatrist.

The ability to manage finances often fades long before more obvious problems arise. I've had patients who've lost houses, who've given hundreds of thousands of dollars to the gardener, who've married their caregiver who drained their bank account. Don't let this happen to your loved one.

People usually retain the ability to make informed health-care choices longer. Still, medical care is complicated, and everyone with dementia eventually loses the ability to make informed health-care choices. It's tragic when an elder doesn't want extraordinary measures taken yet still ends up spending his or her last days in an intensive care unit. It's awful to see a confused person with dementia in the hospital unnecessarily—scared, agitated, and uncomfortable.

Usually, the last capacity to go is what's called testamentary capacity, the ability to make a will, to decide who will get your assets when you're gone. Yet even that ability will fade in most dementia patients. Try to make things clear while you still can. It will avoid legal and financial headaches later, particularly in complicated family situations, such as blended families, those with grown children and second spouses, or when there is disagreement. Ignoring those differences will not make things better.

Look to the Future

Your family may just be reeling from the shock of a dementia diagnosis. But if your elder still retains the capacity to make decisions, now is the time to talk about how to plan for disability benefits, Medicare or Medicaid benefits, and estate planning. As all elders with dementia eventually become disabled in one or more ways, talk about what systems you want in place when that happens. How will Medicare or Medicaid factor into your family's plans? Do the benefits of Medicare or Medicaid differ substantially from the benefits of the health insurance your elder has? If there's a shortfall in those benefits, how will it be bridged? How should the elder's assets be managed while he or she is alive? How will those assets be distributed after the elder dies?

Don't wait to consider these questions. The more you can get done while your loved one can still have a voice, the better.

How to Start the Conversation

Obviously, it's easy to say, "Take action!" It's much more difficult to actually do something. Ideally, we'd set up these systems with our elders before they start to have problems. Alas, that rarely happens. There's no magic way to get financial, health, and legal problems in hand.

Start first by trying to get your elder's cooperation. Explain what worries you. Gently share examples of the kinds of things that you and other family members find concerning. Assure your loved one that you just want to make sure he or she is safe. Try to enlist the help of other family members or friends.

Sometimes, if the elder resists, it helps to point out that accepting a little help now will avoid the possibility of losing all of his or her decision-making rights sooner than necessary. Explain that if you set up systems for health care now, the elder won't have to worry about how decisions will be made when he or she can no longer do so. By making estate plans now, your elder can be sure that his or her wishes will be honored later.

If you wait until a person no longer has decision-making capacity, it is too late to make plans. In that case, your elder and your family will have far fewer options.

If you're lucky enough to be having these conversations while your elder still has adequate mental capacity, be sure to set up systems that can respond to many different situations. Are there family and friends who can help? Who will be in charge of finances? Who will make medical decisions? Who will manage the day-to-day running of the household and the checkbook? When the loved one loses mental capacity, who or what will manage their affairs?

Always try to separate your interests from the interests of your elder. Sometimes they can be very different. If your elder can no longer express his or her wishes, you should try to make decisions based on the elder's beliefs, preferences, and needs.

Shelves of books have been written on estate planning, financial planning, and health-care planning. The goal of this section is simply to give you an overview. You'll definitely need more information and expert advice to craft your family's plan.

Degrees of Control

Whether you need to step in and help your elder with money matters, health-care decisions, or estate planning, there are legal documents, what lawyers call "instruments," that are involved. Some documents give almost unlimited control; others give very limited powers in specific situations. It's important to know the difference so that you can decide what makes the most sense for your family's situation.

Before you decide to grant a relative, an attorney, or a bank these sorts of powers, make sure to check that the person or entity is willing and able to take on these responsibilities. If you're not sure whether the document you have gives you a certain power, call your attorney and check. This will avoid many hassles.

Here are very basic definitions of these documents.

- **Power of Attorney.** This is a legal document that allows a person to appoint someone else to act on his or her behalf. You can limit this power to only apply in certain contexts, most commonly for financial or for health-care decisions. The person who is giving up control is called the principal. The person acting on the principal's behalf is an attorney-in-fact. This doesn't mean that the person actually has to have a law degree, but that they need to act in the principal's best interests at all times. Sometimes this person is also called a proxy. A principal may give this power to one person or to several. A regular power of attorney ends when its purpose is fulfilled or with the incapacity or death of the principal.

A power of attorney may be general, in which the proxy can perform almost any act that the principal might. Or it may be limited, such as for the purpose of selling a piece of property at a particular time. Another variation is durable power of attorney, which remains effective even if the principal becomes incapacitated (see below).

These are powerful documents. They have the potential to give the proxy all the rights and powers of the principal. People with a broad power of attorney can drain a principal's bank account in minutes or sign themselves onto the house title. It's very important to carefully consider who is getting this kind of power.

Be Careful Whom You Trust

An elder couple hired a caregiver without going through an agency for vetting. They gave the caregiver a credit card so she could buy groceries. After a while, the caregiver convinced them to give her durable power of attorney.

The caregiver put checks in front of the couple to sign and drained hundreds of thousands from their estate. She moved most of the furniture out of the house.

When the man fell and broke his hip, the caregiver didn't even take him to the hospital. He lay in bed for months suffering excruciating pain. The caregiver fed the couple TV dinners or, sometimes, spoiled food.

When the evidence finally became so overwhelming that authorities stepped in, the poor man had not only a twisted leg but also a urinary infection and thyroid problems. What's worse, the greater part of the money he and his wife had saved over a lifetime had been stolen.

Don't let this happen to your elder. Before

you give anyone the power to do anything, check and check again. If you don't live locally, make sure that someone visits your elder regularly. Do background investigations. Ask questions. Never allow a caregiver to handle finances. That crosses a line.

- **Durable Power of Attorney.** This works like a plain vanilla power of attorney, but it is durable. That is, it remains in effect if a person becomes incapacitated.

A durable power of attorney for health care differs from a living will in that the attorney-in-fact or the proxy can make decisions *in any situation* in which the person is judged unable to communicate. With a living will, the proxy may only act if the person is permanently unconscious or terminally ill and unable to communicate.

Most important is to find trustworthy people to hold the durable power of attorney for health or financial issues. One woman chose a friend because she did not trust her son. She was right. Several years later, after her dementia had progressed to the point that she was delusional and chairbound, her son took her to his lawyer when her friend was out of town and changed the durable power of attorney to himself, then took over her house and moved her to a dementia facility.

If family members are arguing over who should be in charge or who might have taken advantage, a fiduciary may be the best option for financial issues.

- **Guardianship or Conservatorship.** When a person becomes unable to care for himself or herself, it may become necessary to appoint a person to take care of his or her affairs. This may be called a guardianship or a conservatorship. This requires that social service agencies or the patient's family present evidence before a court that shows that the elder can no longer manage his or her affairs. The court may then appoint a conservator or guardian for the elder, and this person is responsible for making regular reports to the court, showing that everything is being handled legally and in the elder's best interest.

As with a power of attorney, a conservatorship may give broad powers, granting the conservator the power to make any decision involving the elder's life as the conservator for the person and the estate. Or the conservatorship may be limited to a particular task or a particular time period. For instance, a relative might be given the power to handle the sale of a house to pay for the elder's care.

- **Trust.** A trust is a document in which one person transfers money or property to another person for the benefit of a third party. It's also possible for a legal owner to create a trust of property without transferring that property to anyone else. Trusts are governed by the rules and limitations set out in the documents that create them. They're complicated, and you absolutely should seek the advice of an attorney before creating one. Usually, trusts are formed when an estate has enough assets to warrant the extra complexity. Trusts are sometimes overseen by a court, but some types of trusts, like special needs or supplemental needs trusts, which are set up for the benefit of a disabled or mentally ill person, do not require the oversight of a judge.

- **Will.** As everyone knows, this is a document that spells out where a person wants his or her belongings to go after he or she is gone. If the patient has limited assets and a straightforward financial situation, then it may be possible to create a will from standardized documents found on many legal websites. However, if there are significant assets, it's best to consult an attorney.

- **Advance Health-care Directive.** This is a generic term. This document may also be called a living will, a personal directive, an advance directive, or advance decision. It's intended to serve as written instructions outlining what the patient wants to be done medically if he or she becomes unable to make decisions due to illness or incapacity. A living will most commonly leaves medical instructions. Many patients also decide to combine a living will with a durable power of attorney that appoints one person to make health-care decisions if they can't.

It's incredibly important to spell out a patient's wishes when it comes to health-care and end-of-life decisions. End-of-life hospital care can often be unnecessarily prolonged, painful, expensive, and emotionally draining for both patients and their families.

In response to the ever-increasing sophistication of medical care and the often-unhappy outcomes in end-of-life care, the living will was first proposed in 1969. This document has yet to be standardized. Sometimes instructions in a living will fail to fully address the problems and needs of the patient. It's important to carefully consider all possible situations. Gather information about your medical situation from your doctors and caregivers. Make sure to let your friends and family know of your wishes. Because of federal privacy laws, it usually makes sense to name a person who lives nearby to make health-care decisions if necessary.

Sometimes patients and families think that this document simply means "do not treat." Remember that you can spell out both what you want and what you don't want.

Here are some things to consider as you draft your living will.

- Who should make decisions if you're not able to do so? Do you want the same person to make both medical and financial decisions? Or might two different people work better in your situation?

- What medical treatments and care do you want? What treatments frighten you?

- If you stop breathing or your heart stops, do you want to be resuscitated? Unlike the scenes in TV shows and movies, resuscitation of elders works less than 1 percent of the time.

- If you're terminally ill, do you want to remain in the hospital or would you rather be at home?

Once you've drafted your advance directive, make sure you supply a copy to your physicians so that it can be placed in your medical record. Give a copy to your agent, if you've appointed one. Keep a copy in your own files as well.

Remember that the patient can change the directive as long as he or she retains the mental capacity.

Money Matters

Many people think that fiduciaries are all about numbers and documents, but Kim Schwarcz, who specializes in helping elder clients manage their finances, likes interacting with the people. "I treat my clients as if they were my family," she says. "I love working with people."

As with other legal matters, the devil is in the details.

For those with dementia, the ability to manage finances often becomes impaired long before the other symptoms become obvious. While it's best to talk things out with your family before there's a problem, most families don't do this. Too often, when professionals are called in, their main job is to preserve whatever's left of someone's estate, says Schwarcz, who has thirty years in the field.

There are many types of financial management help.

- **Representative payee.** This is a person who is given the power to collect funds such as public assistance, pension, or Social Security payments on behalf of someone who doesn't have the capacity to manage these payments. The dementia facility should never be a Rep Payee.

- **Daily money manager.** You can hire a bookkeeper, an accountant, or a professional agency to handle day-to-day money management for an elder. This person typically makes house calls to help with paying bills, balancing checkbooks, creating budgets, organizing tax records, and filing medical claims. The profession isn't yet regulated, so be sure to do background checks and ask for references. It's good to hire someone who's bonded, or insured, to cover any problems that might arise.

- **Professional fiduciary.** A fiduciary has the responsibility to manage the elder's money only for the elder's benefit. A fiduciary can be the trustee, if a trust is in place. In some states, these professionals are called guardians.

Fiduciaries perform many of the same jobs as daily money managers, but they usually have more training. Fiduciaries may be appointed as conservators, trustees, and representative payees, or attorney to act in financial matters and/or health matters.

In some states, like California, fiduciaries are regulated by the state. There remain huge variations in the training and competence of people who call themselves fiduciaries. Do your due diligence: check references, education, and licensing, if that exists in your state.

• **Estate administrator.** If someone dies without a will, the court will appoint someone to administer the estate. This person's tasks are similar to those of an executor of an estate, but the probate court usually monitors the administrator more closely.

Doing What Works

Often, the solution that makes the most sense doesn't fit into a handy category. For instance, one eighty-five-year-old woman had lost her ability to manage her finances.

She had hired a fiduciary but was adamant about retaining ultimate control over her money.

One day, the fiduciary realized that this woman had lost the ability to write out a check. She couldn't remember where to put the numbers and how to spell them out. So the fiduciary started filling in the payee's name, the amount, and then spelling out the numbers. Then the fiduciary would hand the check to the woman so that she could add the final signature.

In some situations, it might have made sense for this woman to be conserved—that is, for a conservator to handle her affairs completely, with the oversight of a court. In this case, the fiduciary was licensed and bonded. The woman's family lived nearby and kept track of how things were going.

Families need to be careful. They need to keep track. But there are no right answers. Sometimes it makes sense to just do what works.

Final Note

MY MOTHER HAD DEMENTIA, as did my grandmother and my mother-in-law. And in my practice of over twenty years, I have seen over twenty thousand elders with dementia. Every situation is different, but I have included in this guide the main themes affecting areas of care for all elders.

You are not alone. I strongly suggest finding a support group, locally or online, that can encourage, guide, and aid you on this journey.

The most important point is that there are solutions to all the problems that arise. You might not like all the solutions, but they are available. As long as you work for the benefit of your loved one, help them live the life they want (as much as is practically possible), and be available to console and to enjoy moments of joy, you are giving them the greatest gift. If it is not possible to be there in person, then assemble the team that will provide attentive, knowledgeable, timely care with an eye to engagement. A team that will fill the elder's days with meaningful activities and meaningful relationships, and will act in the best interest of the elder's health and finances. Even if you are the primary caregiver, having a team is essential. No one can care for another, especially an elder with dementia, alone. Studies show that caregivers risk serious decline of their own health if they do not have help.

Reading this book and having this information is a giant first step in caring for your loved one. Now, I suggest you go out for a walk. Really. Learning to pace oneself and take time for oneself is job number one for a caregiver. Yes, the elder will need someone else to supervise them while you are gone, but take time for yourself. You will have more energy, empathy, and tolerance for the quirks and demands of dementia care. Care for yourself so you can care for another. It's a cliché because it is true. And when the road ahead seems daunting, remember that you can do this. What a gift you are giving!

Resources and Further Information

ORGANIZATIONS

Administration on Aging Long-Term Care Ombudsman Program

aoa.gov/AoARoot/AoA_Programs/Elder_Rights/
Ombudsman/index.aspx

Advocates nationally for residents of nursing homes, board and care homes, assisted-living facilities, and similar adult care facilities. They work to resolve problems of individual residents and to bring about changes at the local, state, and national levels that will improve residents' care and quality of life.

Administration on Aging Pension Counseling and Information Program

aoa.gov/AoARoot/AoA_Programs/Elder_Rights/
Pension_Counseling/index.aspx

Assists older Americans in accessing information about their retirement benefits and helps them to negotiate with former employers or pension plans for due compensation. The program covers twenty-nine states.

Alliance on Aging

Check your local listings. Most communities have an Alliance on Aging office.

The Alzheimer's Association

www.alz.org

The Alzheimer's Association has chapters throughout the country. It operates referral services, a 24/7 hotline, online communities, newsletters, and links to current research. You can access their five-thousand-volume library online.

Dementia Care Central

www.dementiacarecentral.com/about-us

Resources for dementia caregivers and more. Funded by the National Institutes of Health.

Mayo Clinic Alzheimer's Disease Center

www.mayoclinic.com/health/alzheimers-disease/
   DS00161

In-depth, easy to understand expert overview.

Mayo Clinic Dementia Center

www.mayoclinic.com/health/dementia/DS01131

In-depth, easy to understand expert overview.

National Alliance for Caregiving

www.caregiving.org

Provides information and resources related to family caregiving.

National Association of Professional Geriatric Care Managers

www.caremanager.org

Overview of care management, referrals.

National Center on Elder Abuse

www.ncea.acl.gov

Up-to-date information on research, training, best practices, news, and resources on elder abuse, neglect, and exploitation. It features a state-by-state listing of resources.

National Institute on Aging's Alzheimer's Disease Education and Referral Center

www.nia.nih.gov/alzheimers

Information on research, diagnosis, clinical trials, and government programs and resources.

www.nia.nih.gov/alzheimers/legal-and-financial-issues-people-alzheimers-disease-resource-list

Legal and financial resources list.

Professional Fiduciary Association of California

www.pfac-pro.org

BOOKS

Abbit, Linda. *The Conscious Caregiver*. New York: Adams Media, 2017.

Feil, Naomi. *The Validation Breakthrough*. Baltimore: Health Professions Press, 2012.

Kriseman, Nancy L. *The Mindful Caregiver*. Lanham: Rowman & Littlefield, 2014.

Roche, Lyn. *Coping with Caring*. Harahan: Journey Publications, 2006.

Snyder, Lisa. *Living Your Best Life*. North Branch: Sunrise River Press, 2010.

Williams-Paisley, Kimberly. *Where the Light Gets In*. New York: Crown Archetype, 2016.

CHILDREN'S BOOKS

Bahr, Mary. *The Memory Box*. Park Ridge: Albert Whitman & Company, 1992.

Schnurbush, Barbara. *Striped Shirts and Flowered Pants*. Washington, DC: Magination Press, 2006

Shriver, Maria. *What's Happening to Grandpa?* New York: Little, Brown Books for Young Readers, 2004.

Acknowledgments

Thank you to:

My family, who have put up with me for the last years working endlessly on house calls, developing an education program, and the book.

My team, especially Jane, who has been my Radar O'Reilly to keep me going in the right direction.

Heather, whose grace with words made my work come alive.

Jennifer Chen Tran, my agent, for believing in me when I was not sure, and Denise Silvestro, my editor, who patiently guided me in tucking in all the last details.

Nancy, whose work with the Connected Horse helped me to see that a needed project is worthy of going the extra mile.

The caregivers and thousands of families who have trusted me to work with their suffering elders.

The 3,500 practicing clinical geriatricians who take the extra time to sort out exactly what care is needed and to look at the whole person.

Index